Psychiatry and the Humanities, Volume 1

Associate Editors
Lucie N. Jessner, M.D.
Helm Stierlin, M.D.

Assistant Editor
Gloria H. Parloff

Published under the auspices of the
Forum on Psychiatry and the Humanities
The Washington School of Psychiatry

Psychiatry and the Humanities

VOLUME 1

Editor
Joseph H. Smith, M.D.

New Haven and London   Yale University Press

1976

Designed by John O. C. McCrillis
and set in Baskerville type.
Printed in the United States of America by
The Colonial Press Inc., Clinton, Massachusetts.

Published in Great Britain, Europe, and Africa by
Yale University Press, Ltd., London.
Distributed in Latin America by Kaiman & Polon,
Inc., New York City; in Australasia by Book & Film
Services, Artarmon, N.S.W., Australia;
in Japan by John Weatherhill, Inc., Tokyo.

To Edith Weigert, M.D.

List of Contributors

Sven Arne Bergmann, Fil. Lic.   Lecturer in Swedish, University College, London, 1954–65; Head, Department of Swedish, Munkebäck Senior High School, Göteborg, Sweden

Donald L. Burnham, M.D.   Research Psychiatrist, National Institute of Mental Health; Supervising and Training Analyst, Washington Psychoanalytic Institute; Editor, *Psychiatry*

Louis Dupré, Ph.D.   Professor, Department of Religious Studies, Yale University

Maurice Friedman, Ph.D.   Professor of Religious Studies, Philosophy, and Comparative Literature, San Diego State University; Core Faculty, California School of Professional Psychology

Erich Heller, Ph.D.   Avalon Professor of the Humanities, Northwestern University

Walter Kaufmann, Ph.D.   Professor, Department of Philosophy, Princeton University

Theodore Lidz, M.D.   Professor, Department of Psychiatry, Yale University

Paul Ricoeur, Ph.D.   Professor, Divinity School, University of Chicago; Professor, Université de Nanterre (Paris)

Joseph H. Smith, M.D.   Chairman, Forum on Psychiatry and the Humanities, Washington School of Psychiatry; Teaching Analyst, Washington Psychoanalytic Institute;

Clinical Associate Professor, George Washington University School of Medicine; Consultant, National Institute of Mental Health

Helm Stierlin, M.D., Ph.D. Chief, Abteilung für Psychoanalytische Grundlagenforschung, University of Heidelberg; formerly Acting Chief, Family Studies Section, National Institute of Mental Health; Faculty, Washington Psychoanalytic Institute

Erwin W. Straus, M.D. Clinical Professor of Psychiatry, University of Kentucky; Research Consultant, Veterans Administration, Lexington, Kentucky; deceased, May, 1975

Contents

Preface

Psychiatry and the Humanities, the first in a series of annual volumes, is published under the auspices of The Forum on Psychiatry and the Humanities of The Washington School of Psychiatry. The forum program also includes interdisciplinary seminars, courses, and the annual Edith Weigert lectureship. The initial essay, "Psychoanalysis and the Work of Art," by Paul Ricoeur, was the first of the Weigert lectures, delivered in 1974. The purpose of this annual volume—and also the purpose of each of the other forum activities—is to challenge thought in any one discipline by confrontation with the concepts and methodologies of related disciplines at crucial points of common interest.

In this volume, six humanists and five psychoanalysts engage the issue of interdisciplinary study. Ranging over topics in art, literature, philosophy, language, mysticism, ethics, truth, healing, and creativity, the ten articles that compose the book provide an overview and an introduction to subsequent annual volumes, each of which will be centered on a unitary theme. The first two articles in this volume, those by Paul Ricoeur and Erich Heller, deal directly with aspects of advantage and limitation in applying psychoanalytic study to other fields and in applying the insights and methods of other fields to psychoanalysis. Ricoeur focuses on Freud and art, Heller on Freud and Romanticism. Both articles rigorously demonstrate that there is no easy access to psychoanalysis and, likewise, no easy access to the central problems in the humanities simply by virtue of psychoanalytic training and experience. Ricoeur's profoundly careful reading of the founder of psychoanalysis tells him that Freud was well aware of these difficulties. Heller is not so certain. In any event, both set a standard of scholarship for any interdisciplinary study involving psychoanalytic thought—a standard that is met by the other contributors to this volume and that will remain as a goal for subsequent volumes.

Although the majority of clinician participants in the forum and clinician contributors to this annual are psychoanalysts, and the advancement of psychoanalytic theory is one of the nodal points upon which our efforts converge, we have chosen *psychiatry* as the generically proper term in our title. However, the psychiatry we have in mind is not only a psychiatry that includes psychoanalysis but also a psychiatry that has been fundamentally "renovated"—to use a term of Ricoeur's—by psychoanalysis. In this sense, psychiatry, and not just psycho-analysis, aims for as full as possible a self-knowledge of one's past, present, and envisioned future. The various methods of therapeutic intervention are properly determined not by virtue of variation from this aim, but by the condition of the patient at the point of therapeutic encounter.

In pursuing his clinical goal, the psychiatrist inevitably considers the humanist's exposition of what man has thought and done about the problems and rewards of his existence. At the same time, the psychiatrist's sensitivity to the pressures and stimuli that help to shape thought, will, affects, and imagina-tion can deepen the humanist's understanding of why and how man has responded as he has to the mysteries that confront him.

It is preeminently appropriate that this initial volume of the annual should be dedicated to Edith Weigert, as a Festschrift in honor of her eightieth birthday. During the course of Dr. Weigert's long, distinguished, and productive career, the overlapping interests of the psychiatrist and the humanist have always been of deep concern to her.

Edith Weigert received her medical and psychoanalytic

training in Germany, where she was born, spent five years on
the staff of the neuropsychiatric department of the University
Medical School of Berlin, and in 1929 became an assistant to
Dr. Ernst Simmel at the first German psychoanalytic hospital
in Berlin-Tegel. As a member of the Berlin Psychoanalytic
Institute, she was a participant in the discussions led by
Abraham, Sachs, Alexander, Glover, Melanie Klein, Frieda
Fromm-Reichmann, Fenichel, and many others. But the
political pressures of Nazi Germany became too ominous, and
she left, spending four years in Turkey before coming to the
United States in 1938. Here she joined those immigrants from
Europe who have so greatly vitalized and enriched psychoanalysis and psychiatry in this country. She entered the private
practice of psychoanalysis, but always devoted a large portion
of her time to investigation and writing, and also entered
actively into the life of the psychiatric educational community.
Along with Harry Stack Sullivan, Frieda Fromm-Reichmann,
and their colleagues, she had a leading role in the development of the Washington School of Psychiatry. From 1944 to
1946 she was president of the Washington-Baltimore Psychoanalytic Society, from 1945 to 1954 chairman of the Education
Committee of the Washington Psychoanalytic Institute, and
from 1963 to 1974 chairman of the faculty of the Washington
School of Psychiatry. She has also been a major influence in
the establishment of the Forum on Psychiatry and the
Humanities.

The many contributions she has made to psychoanalytic
literature represent a creative synthesis, always transcending
the viewpoint of any particular school, and often of psychoanalysis proper. Her articles explicating or reflecting the
thought of Kierkegaard, Husserl, Heidegger, Sartre, Jaspers,
Buber, and Tillich have been of major importance in introducing phenomenological and existential thought into American psychiatry and psychoanalysis. However, she is most
clearly present in those articles which directly convey her own

views of what is essential in human existence and how a grasp of these essentials can guide the healing process.

"The courage to love," she wrote in her book, "does not deny the tragedies of human existence in manic flight reactions. The courage to love endures the distress of disillusionment and frustration, faces the anxiety of loneliness in the labor of mourning. The courage to love is inexhaustible in its resources of genuine repentance, repair, and reconciliation, since this courage enables man to trust without rational proof in the dignity and wholeness of the I and the Thou, not as partial objects and means of only sensual, and therefore egocentric, gratification, but this courage trusts in the creative wholeness of the We." *

J.H.S.

* *The Courage to Love* (New Haven: Yale University Press, 1970), p. 34.

Acknowledgments

The Forum on Psychiatry and the Humanities and this publication have been instituted with the crucial support of Robert G. Kvarnes, Irving M. Ryckoff, Eugene Meyer, Seymour S. Mintz, Leon Gerber, Alvin I. Brown, Thomas Allen, Wolfgang Weigert, James Gutmann, Barbara B. Peake, and the many other friends, colleagues, and students of Edith Weigert who participated in the establishment of the annual Edith Weigert Lecture.

The editors also wish to express special thanks to Katherine S. Henry for her assistance in the preparation of the manuscript.

Psychiatry, Art, and Literature

Psychiatry and the Humanities, Volume 1

1

Psychoanalysis and the Work of Art*

PAUL RICOEUR

Opponents of psychoanalysis concur in reproaching it for *reducing* art and esthetic creation. An attentive reader of Freud's writings should instead, it seems to me, puzzle over Freud's modesty, his protests of incompetence, his admissions of failure, and, finally, his insistence on stressing the limits of psychoanalysis when applied to art.

Such warnings abound in the last chapter of *Leonardo da Vinci and a Memory of his Childhood*: pathography, it is stated, does not propose to explain the great man's work, and of course no one can be reproached for not delivering what was never promised. The proposed goal lies in explaining Leonardo's inhibitions in his sexual life and in his artistic activity. As for the artist's talent and his capacity for work, these are too intimately tied to sublimation. For this reason we must admit that the essence of the artistic function must remain psychoanalytically inaccessible to us. In short, if psychoanalysis does not explain to us why Leonardo was an artist, it at least allows us to capture the manifestations and the limits of his art.

These are not merely isolated reservations; they are found in *An Autobiographical Study*, in *Civilization and its Discontents*, in the *Outline of Psycho-Analysis*. It is repeatedly asserted in various

* The Edith Weigert Lecture, sponsored by the Forum on Psychiatry and the Humanities, Washington School of Psychiatry, Oct. 10, 1974.

forms that the esthetic evaluation of a work of art as well as an explanation of artistic talent are not psychoanalytic tasks.

These persistent cautions should make us think.[1] My investigation aims at measuring their true importance. My inquiry will concern the hypothesis that the admission of an inherent limit in applying psychoanalysis to art is purely tactical and serves only to lower the resistances of a listener or a reader unfamiliar with psychoanalysis to an explanation which, in fact, leaves *no remainder.* I would like to show the insufficiencies of arguments supporting this thesis and to seek in Freud's own metapsychoanalysis the reasons for his scruples. I shall thus not consider arguments foreign to Freud's own work but shall continue to limit myself to an internal approach.

An initial argument could perhaps be drawn from the *strategic* function performed by elements borrowed from art in the most incontestable of psychoanalytic works, *The Interpretation of Dreams.* Far from being constituted without any reference to works of art and then being "applied" to them later, for psychoanalysis the comparison between dreams, symptoms, folktales, and myths is absolutely primitive and organically tied to the central demonstration of the *Traumdeutung.* This parallelism is astonishing indeed: from the outset, Freud's fundamental discovery in his self-analysis is placed under the aegis of a hero of Greek legend whose existence is, for us, purely *literary.* Oedipus exists only in *Oedipus Rex,* a character drawn by Sophocles and nothing more. In this way,

---

1. Do not the introductory declarations of "The Moses of Michelangelo," which, we must not forget, was first published anonymously, refer to the same caution? "I may say at once that I am no connoisseur in art, but simply a layman. I have often observed that the subject-matter of works of art has a stronger attraction for me than their formal and technical qualities, though to the artist their value lies first and foremost in these latter. I am unable rightly to appreciate many of the methods used and the effects obtained in art. I state this so as to secure the reader's indulgence for the attempt I propose to make here."

an individual drama is at once identified and named through the mediation of a figure which poetry first set up as a mythical paradigm. Of course, it is not the poetic, literary, esthetic aspect of the figure of Oedipus that fascinated Freud, but the "subject-matter" and the identical nature of the *content* signified by the myth and that revealed by self-analysis. One properly esthetic feature, at least, is pertinent: the universality which belongs to literary fiction. So if the myth is not dealt with as fiction, its sense content nevertheless presents a specific feature which permits a *particular* psychological fact to bear directly the seal of a universal structure. This is expressed in the very name given to the experience discovered along the strict path of self-analysis; thereafter the experience will bear a Greek name.[2]

Now this demonstrative schema functions only if, implicitly, one grants that the work of art has the same explanation as the dream. Or, more precisely, it is necessary that dreams and works of art be reciprocally paradigmatic in a demonstration that is rigorously circular. This is possible if they occupy the role of model from different points of view: the dream, from a genetic point of view; the work of art, from a structural point of view.

Indeed, on the one hand dream analysis provides the key for interpreting the derivation of meaning, in accordance with the formula that gives chapter 3 of *The Interpretation of Dreams* its

2. The letters to Fliess attest to the primitive origins of this parallelism: "One single thought of general value has been revealed to me. I have found, in my own case too, falling in love with the mother and jealousy of the father, and I now regard it as a universal event of early childhood. . . . If that is so, we can understand the riveting power of *Oedipus Rex*, in spite of all the objections raised by reason against its presupposition of destiny; and we can understand why the later 'dramas of destiny' were bound to fail so miserably. . . . Each member of the audience was once, in germ and in phantasy, just such an Oedipus, and each one recoils in horror from the dream-fulfilment here transplanted into reality, with the whole quota of repression which separates his infantile state from his present one" (Letter to Fliess, Oct. 15, 1897, *Standard Edition* 1:265. Hereafter referred to as *S.E.*).

title: "a dream is the fulfilment of a wish" (*S.E.*, 4:122). The formula itself summarizes a series of propositions: dreams have a meaning; this meaning calls for a precise type of decoding, detail by detail; the latent meaning is separated from the apparent meaning by a work—the "dream-work"—which gathers together the relations of force and the relations of meaning, as is expressed in the notions of displacement, condensation, representability, secondary revision; and finally, desires represented in dreams in a disguised manner are the oldest desires, archaic and infantile.

This is what is paradigmatic in dreams and this is what is analogically transposed from the dream to the work of art.

The *structural* aspect, however, is no less important than the *genetic* aspect. One could neither identify nor name a mental production, if one were not able to detect an invariable to serve as a prime analogon for its diverse variants. It is here that the work of art provides an exemplarity all its own: if self-analysis revealed the "riveting power," the "compulsion" of the Greek legend, in its turn the elevation of the intimate personal complex to the level of poetic fiction increased the seal of universality on an experience that would otherwise remain particular, incommunicable, and ultimately silent. The individual *secret* is a universal *fate;* for this reason, it can be *stated.* It has *already* been stated.

What is at stake in this circular relation is thus much more than the possibility of articulating a theory of culture based on the semantics of desire;[3] it is the possibility of rendering the

3. It is this aspect that I developed in *Freud and Philosophy*, part 2, "The Interpretation of Culture," in the section titled "The Analogy of the Work of Art" (pp. 163–77). This is why the passage to institutions and, with this, the ethical character that becomes part of this universal fate, are strongly emphasized here. The connection between ontogenesis and phylogenesis appeared to me in particular as a means of proving that psychoanalysis is from the outset a theory of culture, because its object is not brute wishes but wishes in a cultural setting. In the present essay, I should like to return to an even more primitive problem, which concerns the very intelligibility of analytic experience. This is why I have insisted on the *structural* function of literary fiction in relation to the *genetic* function of analytic interpretation.

genesis itself *intelligible.* The *Three Essays on Sexuality* reveal the fundamentally "historical" aspect of human sexuality, tied to the successive constitutions by which it passes from "stage" to "stage." This "historicity"—which the theory of stages will continue to develop in the course of successive editions of the *Three Essays*—holds within it a serious threat to the *scientific* character of psychoanalysis. How could the "history" of desire be told if it were not set into *forms* capable of being fixed in cultural denominations? Genesis must then indeed be based on structure if it is to be an explanation, that is, if it is to make us understand.

This can be shown by a careful study of the instances of literary examples in the *Traumdeutung.* Literary fictions—and among them, the Oedipus tragedy—are evoked in reference to a very special category of dreams, which Freud calls "typical dreams" (*S.E.*, 4:241 ff.). Among these dreams of universal signification, Freud cites dreams of nudity and exhibition and dreams of the death of close relatives. Unlike the dreams analyzed in the earlier sections, which Freud says constitute a dream-world constructed by each person "according to his individual peculiarities and so to make it unintelligible to other people," these dreams have "the same meaning for everyone" (p. 241). Now these are also dreams where the associative method proves particularly inadequate and sterile. It is precisely for these dreams that literature offers a schema of meaning, a sort of doublecheck *easier to read* than the dream itself.

This is possible because the forces of inhibition which are responsible for distorting the dream have been partially eliminated in the literary work for reasons that will be apparent later. This is true in the case of Hans Christian Andersen's story *The Emperor's New Clothes,* which provides a less distorted version of the dream of nudity with its apparent bizarre characteristics.[4] And as the myth of Paradise, where

4. Speaking of dreams of nakedness, where the dreamer is embarrassed and the spectators are strangely indifferent, Freud observes: "We possess an interesting piece

Adam and Eve are naked, has the same root meaning, and since, on the other hand, the fantasy itself appears naked in the perversion termed *exhibitionism*, a series can be formed from dreams, folktales, myths, and symptoms. This series is structured by the invariable which we call "typical" dreams and which also forms *the* meaning of the tale, of the myth, and of the symptom. We shall return later to an important aspect of the structure, namely, the fact that the invariable is nothing other than the cross-reference from one variant to the other: dream, symptom, myth, tale. For the present, let us content ourselves with recognizing the way in which the genesis is reinforced by the structure through the mediation of poetic fiction.[5]

Indeed, it is this very reciprocal relation between individual genesis and universal type which permits the connecting of dreams of the death of a close relative, dreams accompanied by deep grief, to the Oedipus legend. Before he even mentions Sophocles' tragedy, Freud insists on "the obscure information which is brought to us by mythology and legend from the primaeval ages of human society" (*S.E.,* 4:256). Out of this obscure information there progressively appears "an unpleasing picture of the father's despotic powers and of the ruthlessness with which he made use of it. Kronos devoured his children, just as the wild boar devours the sow's litter; while

---

of evidence that the dream in the form in which it appears—partly distorted by wish-fulfilment—has not been rightly understood. For it has become the basis *[die Grundlage]* of a fairy tale which is familiar to us all in Hans Andersen's version, *The Emperor's New Clothes*" (*S.E.,* 4:243).

5. Freud is content to note: "There can be no doubt that the connections between our typical dreams and fairy tales and the material of other kinds of creative writing are neither few nor accidental. It sometimes happens that the sharp eye of a creative writer has an analytic realization of the process of transformation of which he is habitually no more than the tool. If so, he may follow the process in a reverse direction and so trace back the imaginative writing to a dream" (*S.E.,* 4:246). In the same way, the legend of Odysseus appearing naked in the eyes of Nausicaä and her maidens is transposed into a common dream by Gottfried Keller in *Der grüne Heinrich* (ibid.).

Zeus emasculated his father and made himself ruler in his place" (p. 256).

Freud is able to pass from this mythological notation to the analysis of some death dreams of adult neurotics in analysis. And this is because, for him, there is no line of demarcation between the normal and the pathological. At the most, he asserts that neurotics present "on a magnified scale" (p. 261) the same feelings of love and hate as do most children. This is why one can follow the inverse path, from the symptom toward the legend: "This discovery is confirmed by a legend that has come down to us from classical antiquity: a legend whose profound and universal power to move can only be understood if the hypothesis I have put forward in regard to the psychology of children has an equally universal validity. What I have in mind is the legend of King Oedipus and Sophocles' drama which bears his name" (p. 261).

It is thus the psychology of children that furnishes the core of the argument, provided that it has "universal validity." But it is the legend and its literary elaboration which provide the evidence for this. The explanation is thus perfectly circular: psychoanalysis brings out "the particular nature of the material"—which a bit further on is called "the primaeval dream-material"; but it is the tragedy which makes it speak: "There must be something which makes a voice within us ready to recognize the compelling force of destiny in the *Oedipus*. . . . His destiny moves us only because it might have been ours—because the oracle laid the same curse upon us before our birth as upon him. . . . Our dreams convince us that that is so" (p. 262). The drama's superiority in regard to dreams consists only in that it "shows" us our desires as they are both realized and punished. But the drama, in its turn, can be traced back to the dream, as was the case in the Andersen fairy tale. In Sophocles' tragedy itself the myth's meaning is mirrored in a dream which occurs as a quotation; Jocasta herself consoles Oedipus with these words:

Many a man ere now in dreams has lain
With her who bare him. He hath least annoy
Who with such omens troubleth not his mind

> [Lewis Campbell translation,
> ll. 982 ff., quoted in
> *S.E.* 4:264]

But the role of literary fiction is not only that of revealing the universality of a structure; it also allows us to specify in what the structural *invariable* consists. It is not an eternal essence but the law governing a series, the law of constructing cross-references from one variant to the other. We have already seen, in connection with the "typical" dream of nudity, how the meaning of the dream was repeated in different ways in the fairy tale, the myth, and in the perverse symptom. Even within the sphere of fiction the same cross-reference occurs: the "type" signified by a dream refers to various poetic creations which can be arranged according to a scale of distortion, following the degree to which repression has altered the basic readability. In this way, the structural kinship between *Hamlet* and *Oedipus*, perceived as early as the period of the letters to Fliess, is founded at once on the identity "of the same material" and on "the whole difference in the mental life of these two widely separated epochs of civilization: the secular advance of repression in the emotional life of mankind." In *Oedipus Rex*, the infantile fantasy "is brought into the open and realized as it would be in a dream" (*S.E.*, 4:264). In *Hamlet*, the repression is so accentuated that it is only from the hero's inhibitions that one can then move back to the Oedipal core—namely, that Hamlet is unable to accomplish the prescribed vengeance "on the man who did away with his father and took that father's place with his mother, this man who shows him the repressed wishes of his own childhood realized" (p. 265).

It is not the accuracy of Freud's interpretation of *Hamlet* that

I am concerned with here, but rather its strategic function in his demonstration. It aims at strengthening the invariability of the "type" by relating the difference in regard to another version of the *same* symbol to forces which cause the identity of signification to be dispersed under various disguises. At the same time, this identity exists nowhere but in the correlation, not only of the dream fantasy and the literary drama but also of different cultural expressions of the same theme.

It is this *thematic* unity of works of art, dreams, and symptoms that gives the present argument its force and inclines one to consider Freud's scruples, mentioned earlier in this essay, to be only simulated. The strict parallelism implied in the circular argumentation of the *Traumdeutung* renders plausible indeed the suspicion that Freud's reservations are only a clever maneuver directed against the resistances of a nonanalytic public.

However, this argument is not itself decisive. And this for an important reason. The purely strategic—and if one may say so, simply *apologetic*—use of literary examples, of poetic fictions, in a work statedly dealing with the interpretation of dreams, precisely excludes treating cultural works according to their specific nature, that is, as artistic creations. Quite the opposite, only their libidinal origin is taken into consideration, what above we called the "material" *(Rohstoff)*, "the primaeval dream-material" from which the legend arose. Now Freud's scruples, we remember, concerned the formal and esthetic qualities of the work as a creation. One thus cannot confine oneself to the first argument.

A second argument against the real sincerity of Freud's modest claims in regard to the application of psychoanalysis to art can be drawn from the few studies in which works of art no longer serve only as supporting examples but are analyzed in themselves. These essays seem to justify the assertion that these works are *analogues* to dreams and to symptoms and that the analogy itself is based in the *fantasmatic structure* common to the series of analogues. Indeed, the analogy is not a vague resemblance but a constructed kinship.

Let us see, then, how Freud marks out what I shall call the *space of fantasy* in general and distributes the figures of fantasy within this homogeneous sphere.

The short essay *Der Dichter und das Phantasieren* (1908), translated into English under the title "Creative Writers and Day-dreaming" (*S.E.*, vol. 9), prepares the reader for this unitary vision of the entire field of *das Phantasieren* by ordering along a graduated scale diverse mental productions, whose extreme forms seem to lack any common measure: fantasies of the dreamer and of the neurotic at one end of the spectrum; poetic creations, which the layman attributes to a "separate personality," at the other end of the spectrum. The distance between them can be reduced if one can insert suitable intermediaries between the opposing terms. This is the tactic employed by this clever little essay. The intermediary degrees considered here are children's *games* and adult's *day-dreams* (*Tagträume*). Then come folktales, where the hero portrays "His Majesty the Ego, the hero alike of every day-dream and of every story" (*S.E.*, 9:150). Then come psychological novels, which are related to the egocentric type by a series of gradual transitions until one reaches the point where the author appears to be the spectator of his characters' actions. The continuity of these transitions allows the extension, step by step, of the model of *Wunscherfüllung* (wish-fulfillment) provided by the interpretation of dreams.

The critical difference between the work of art and the fantasy does not, in fact, reside in the instinctual "material" (*Rohstoff*) employed but in the *technique* by means of which the writer obtains the *effect* produced on his reader. While the day-dream causes only shame in the dreamer and makes him tend to hide his fantasies from others, the artist creates pleasure out of what should repel us or leave us cold. How? All *ars poetica,* Freud tells us, is contained in the techniques by which the artist manages to *seduce* us by offering us an "increment of pleasure," a purely *formal* pleasure, belonging to the very representation of fantasies. This "incitement premium"—technically termed "fore-pleasure"—allows us to take pleasure in the liberation of psychic forces which find their fantasmatic expression in the work. "We give the name of an *incentive bonus,* or a *fore-pleasure,* to a yield of pleasure such as this, which is offered to us so as to make possible the release of still greater pleasure arising from deeper psychical sources" (*S.E.,* 9:153).

This distinction between the thematical and the technical allows the difference between fantasy and the work of art to be included inside the sphere of the *Phantasieren* (which I am calling here "fantasy in general"). And this distinction does not cast "technique" outside the space of fantasy, to the extent that the theory of "fore-pleasure" itself arises out of the common *economy* which presides over the release of tensions coming from the unconscious sphere, which will later be called the "Id." But, as early as the *Three Essays on Sexuality,* the theory of the "incitement premium" is solidly anchored in the first theory of instinctual drives. As in the series of maneuvers that bring the complete sexual act to its term, so esthetic pleasure serves to set off deep-seated releases. This connection between the technical and the hedonistic thus maintains the work of art within the sphere of wish-fulfillment. At the same time, it reveals what is essential in Freud's strategy as he confronts the great enigma of creativity. Unable to be worked out as a whole, it is dissolved bit by bit. After isolating the thematic, one steps around the obstacle of creation by replacing it with the question of the *effect* produced on the art lover, and one links the technique to the effect of pleasure. The problem is thus kept within the limits of an economy of desire.

It was in *Jokes and their Relation to the Unconscious* (1905) that Freud first transposed from the theory of instinctual drives to

esthetics his concept of the economy of fore-pleasure. Jokes
indeed have the advantage of presenting for analysis a precise
pleasure-effect, for it is pinpointed by the release of laughter.
As such the purely *verbal* techniques of *Witz* present nothing
strikingly new in regard to what the analysis of the dream-
work had brought to light: condensation, displacement, representation by the contrary, etc.; nothing new except an
emphasis that the very notion of "dream-work" did not allow
to be foreseen, in the sense of a correspondence between these
procedures and figures of rhetoric. This somewhat linguistical
interpretation of the "distortion" performed by the dream-
work unquestionably allows the entire field of verbal productions to be annexed to the domain of fantasy.

But it is in particular by reason of its contribution to an
economic theory of laughter that the essay on *Witz* assures the
continuity among all the phenomena belonging to the space of
fantasy. The pure technique of words, characteristic of *Witz*,
gives the mind a surface pleasure which serves as a release for
forces that are hidden in the obscene, aggressive, or cynical
modalities of word play. The pleasure taken in word play, as a
work on the body of the word, is in itself a minimal pleasure,
tied to the saving of psychic work which is realized in
condensation, displacement, etc. In this way, the pleasure
derived from nonsense frees us from the restrictions that logic
inflicts on our thought and lightens the yoke of all intellectual
pursuits. But if this pleasure is minimal, as are the savings it
expresses, it still has the remarkable power of contributing, in
the form of a bonus, to the erotic, aggressive, or skeptical
tendencies.

The puzzle of esthetic *technique* fades away if it is considered
not from the perspective of the creator but from that of the
effect produced on the public. At the same time, this weakens
the objection that could be drawn from the fact that the
author cannot be submitted to analytic investigation because
he is unable to contribute by his associations—in particular by

the work of transference—to clarifying the energies freed by
his own imaginative creation. For if the author is beyond our
reach, the layman who experiences the pleasure-effect produced by the work of art *is* accessible to analytic investigation.
He is in the position of the nocturnal dreamer and of the
day-dreamer.

Once the space of fantasy has been delimited by this initial
work of circumscription, it is then possible to determine the
features of the fantastic that guarantee the homogeneity of the
phenomena placed under this common heading. I should like
to stress two of these features which, in Freud's work,
determine *Phantasieren* in its very essence.

The first is discussed within the framework of the *Dream-
work*, in chapter 6 of the *Traumdeutung*, under the heading
"Considerations of Representability" (*Rücksicht auf Darstellbarkeit; S.E.,* 5:339 ff.). It is the third operation of the dream-work,
after condensation and displacement. This operation consists
in substituting for a verbal expression of a given thought a
"pictorial" expression. But the sense of this *Darstellbarkeit*
exceeds representability in visual images, for it extends to
verbal images themselves, which, by reason of this figurative
capacity, are restored to their full polysemic resources and to
the entire range of their ambiguities. This causes Freud to say
that language is here carried back to the ancient richness of
hieroglyphic writing.[6] This representability—something like
an aptitude for *staging*—is treated elsewhere under the title of
"formal" regression (in order to distinguish it from "temporal"
regression and "topological" regression);[7] that is, it is treated
as the regression of logical links moving toward concrete and

6. "Yet, in spite of all this ambiguity, it is fair to say that the productions of the
dream-work, which, it must be remembered, *are not made with the intention of being
understood,* present no greater difficulties to their translators than do the ancient
hieroglyphic scripts to those who seek to read them" (*The Interpretation of Dreams, S.E.,*
5:341).
7. *The Interpretation of Dreams, S.E.,* 5:548.

figurative expression. Its kinship with hieroglyphic writing allows us, in turn, to extend to the nonverbal aspects of dreams a notion of "text," the entire field of what is representable. It is this "textual" aspect, in the extended sense of the word, that is implied when we apply to dreams, in all of their figurative aspects, the metaphor of censorship, whose meaning first refers to the "blotting out" of correspondence, newspapers, and texts in general by a political authority with an essentially repressive function. Representability, however, attests to the *nonverbal* character of the dream-work, even in its properly verbal expressions. When the dream-work utilizes language, it continues to be nonverbal to the extent that its writing is more hieroglyphic than phonetic.

This nonverbal or preverbal character of the *figurative text* of dreams explains the ease with which one can, without leaving the space of *figurative* fantasy, move to plastic expressions, as, for instance, in the case of examples borrowed from *statuary*.

We find this in the essay "The Moses of Michelangelo" (1914; *S.E.,* 13:211–36). The marble statue of Moses, erected by Michelangelo in the church of San Pietro in Vincoli in Rome, is treated in this way as a fantasy objectified in stone. The puzzle it offers to our understanding and the effect it produces on our sensibilities are treated *as* the enigma and the affective effect that a dream would produce in the sort of "staging" that is its own. In both cases, it is the "intention" of the artist and of the dreamer that is to be discovered by way of analysis. "To discover his intention, though, I must first find out the meaning and content of what is represented in his work; I must, in other words, be able to *interpret* it" (p. 212). The work of stone and the work of words (and it is not by chance that *Hamlet* is evoked once more in this context), to the extent that they are different modalities of the same fundamental *representability,* give rise to the same need—"the need of discovering in it some source of power beyond them [the impressive thoughts and the splendor of language] alone" (p. 213).

It is thus not surprising that a statue may be treated exactly *like* a dream. In both cases interpretation involves the same attention to unnoticed *details,* the same sort of separate treatment—analytic in the strict sense of the word—of each of these details taken in themselves, especially those that are disregarded or ignored ("the rubbish-heap, as it were, of our observations," p. 222). This is true of the position of the *Moses'* right-hand finger in relation to the draping of his beard, the position of the tablets of the Law upside down and balancing on an edge. In this way, little by little, the figure of a compromise is drawn between opposing movements that took place the instant *before* and of which there remain only vestiges in the present position: "What we see before us is not the inception of a violent action but the remains of a movement that has already taken place" (p. 229). What follows in the essay confirms that the statue can and must be deciphered like a "text"; Freud returns here to a written text, the Book of Exodus, in order to measure the *difference* between Michelangelo's stone-text and that of Scripture. The sense of Michelangelo's work lies in the difference between the two texts, one depicting the hero in the throes of violent anger, the other daring to create "a different Moses . . . one superior to the historical or traditional Moses" (p. 233).

Moreover, the interpretation can go so far as to understand the realization, not only in terms of its difference in regard to an earlier textual and scriptural model, but its difference in regard to the *idea* that analysis reconstructs. Freud hazards this conclusion: "In his creations Michelangelo has often enough gone to the utmost limit of what is expressible in art; and perhaps in his statue of Moses he has not completely succeeded, if his purpose *[seine Absicht]* was to make the passage of a violent gust of passion visible in the signs left behind it in the ensuing calm" (p. 236). Moving back in this way from the realization to the intention, analysis can retranslate the intention into *words* ("But why should the artist's intention not be capable of being communicated and comprehended in *words,* like any other fact of mental life?" p. 212). It is this *verbal* translation of a *plastic* figure that emerges in the summary words of the essay: "And so he carved his Moses on the Pope's tomb, not without a reproach against the dead pontiff, as a warning to himself, thus, in self-criticism, rising superior to his own nature" (p. 234).

These successive translations from writing into a message in stone, and then again from stone into discourse, are produced within the same space of fantasy on the basis of the representability common to its various expressions.

This last remark leads us to the second characteristic of the fantastic as such, which founds the analogy of its various incarnations. This is its character of being basically *substitutive,* that is, a sign's capacity to hold for, to take the place of, to replace something else.

This substitutive character is implied in the psychoanalytic notion of "sense"; to say that dreams have "sense" is not to designate what they mean in appearance but to point to the latent sense that is to be reconstructed from them. This is why it is necessary to interpret: "for 'interpreting' a dream implies assigning a 'meaning' to it—that is, replacing *[ersetzen]* it by something which fits into the chain of our mental acts as a link having a validity and importance equal to the rest" (*Interpretation of Dreams,* in *S.E.,* 4:96). Interpretation, though, does no more than follow the inverse route of that taken by the dream-*work.* The latter fulfills a wish only by dissimulating its object under a *substituted* object. For this reason, the symptomatic value of dreams is due entirely to the absolutely primitive *substitutability* of the *sign-effect.* Transposition, deformation, distortion—all effects that are included in the German expression *Traumentstellung* ("distortion" in English)—are grounded in this capacity of signs to replace something else, and, in particular, other signs. The relation hiding-showing, which is essential to the idea of "the disguised fulfillment of a repressed wish," is a result of this relation of substitution by which the "same" sense is preserved in the "other" sense. Displacement and condensation are only the mechanisms by which substitution itself renders itself unrecognizable, without canceling the chain of meanings. And the whole analytic maneuver is built upon a substitution in the opposite direction: how, Freud asks at the beginning of the essay on "The Unconscious," do we arrive at knowledge of the unconscious? His answer: "It is of course only as something conscious that we know it, after it has undergone transformation *[Umsetzung]* or translation *[Übersetzung]* into something conscious" (*S.E.,* 14:166).

Substitution takes on the precise form given to it by psychoanalysis when it is combined with the preceding feature, *staging,* which is essential to the representability of dreams. More precisely, it is when dreams refer back to some *infantile scene* that representability and substitutability combine their effects: "On this view a dream might be described as a *substitute [Ersatz] for an infantile scene modified by being transferred on to a recent experience.* The infantile scene is unable to bring about its own revival and has to be content with returning as a dream" (*The Interpretation of Dreams, S.E.,* 5:546).

In the representable-substitutable character of fantasies, we grasp the most important feature of the Freudian "fantastic." The most primitive possibility of the work of art is contained in this discovery, at first disconcerting, that we are never dealing with signs that would give us the thing itself, but with signs that are already signs of signs.

In order to understand this, we must go back to what Freud calls *primal* repression, which means that every observable repression, to which we are able to relate this or that distortion, is already a subsequent repression, "after the fact" *(nachträglich)* in relation to the *Urverdrängung* that is always posited behind repression "proper" *(eigentlich)*. Because of this, we never witness an initial substitution, and analysis is compelled to move among signs of signs. Of course, psychoanalysis must posit at the level of *theoretical* concepts, and consequently at the level of metapsychological construction, something like an initial psychic "presentation" of drives, primordial holding for. In his writings on metapsychology, Freud creates to this end the concept of *Repräsentanz*—a technical term, translated as *Presentation* (*Representation* in the *Standard Edition*). At the beginning of the essay on "The Unconscious," we read: "We have learnt from psycho-analysis that the essence of the process of repression lies, not in putting an end to, in annihilating, the idea which represents an instinct *[den Trieb repräsentierende Vorstellung]*, but in preventing it from becoming conscious" (*S.E.*, 14:166).

This absolutely primitive linking of force and sense is presupposed by all "transpositions" and all "translations" from the unconscious to the conscious. But it is presupposed only as a theoretical construction which allows psycho-*analysis* to be a *psycho*-analysis, that is, to always deal not with instincts—presumed biological realities—but with the "representatives of instinct," whether these representatives be "ideas" or "affects." The decisive fact is that psychoanalysis moves, has always moved, among the "mental derivatives *[psychische Abkömenlinge]* of the repressed representative" (*S.E.*, 14:148). The notion of primal repression is there to remind us that we are always in the mediate, in the already expressed, the already said: "The second stage of repression, *repression proper,* affects mental derivatives of the repressed representative, or such trains of thought *[Gedankenzüge]* as, originating elsewhere, have come into associative connection with it" (*S.E.*, 14:148).

It is thus because analysis knows only secondary distortions that it also knows only signs of signs. Communication between the systems Ucs., Pcs., Cs., can only be deciphered inside the signifying architecture of the derivatives: "In brief, it must be said that the *Ucs.* is continued into *[stezt sich in]* what are known as derivatives" (*S.E.*, 14:190). "Formation substitutives," "symptoms," "return of the repressed" are so many different *vicissitudes* which guide the game of substitutions. The possible combinations revealed here are immense; among the "derivatives" of the *Ucs.*, some present at the same time the superior organization of the system *Cs.* and the specific laws of the *Ucs.* system. These hybrid formations we know well: they are the fantasies of the normal individual and of the neurotic, but they are also the highly complex substitutive formations with which the artist *plays*.

If we apply these remarks from metapsychology to the notion of psychic text offered above, then it must be said that psychoanalysis knows only "translations" of texts, different versions which come from no original text. Being in some sense primitive, substitution is the very fabric of the "fantastic."

In this respect, so-called childhood memories provide the best example of this fantastic constitution, and prefigure works of fiction. The very expression "infantile scene," which we borrowed earlier from the *Traumdeutung*, expresses the twofold character of representability and distortion in the very play of theatrical exposition. Nothing demonstrates better what the fantasy's construction "after the fact" consists of than does the "screen-memory." By its character of being already substituted, memory belongs to the "fantastic." One sees that poetic imagination has no need to be grafted onto memory; it is already at work there. Between *Dichten* and *Phantasieren* the link is absolutely primitive.

On the basis of this analysis, one sees the position that can be taken *against* the irreducibility of the work of art. The same interplay of representability and substitution which is already functioning in dreams and memory continues in esthetics. Is this not what was presupposed a bit earlier by the work of interpretation when it *referred back* from a dream to a fairy tale, from a fairy tale to a myth, in order to go back to a perverse symptom? Was not this cross-reference from one level to the other based upon the eminently substitutable character of fantasy in general? Furthermore, is not the deciphering itself entirely reducible to this interplay of references?

There is no doubt that this is one of the most decisive implications of Freudian fantasy in regard to the theory of art. The possibility of treating a work of art *as* a dream is based on the possibility of *substituting* one for the other. The admirable short essay, *"Das Unheimliche"* (1919)—"The 'Uncanny' "— describes, in this respect, the ultimate consequences of the absolutely homogeneous nature of the fantastic resulting from the mutual substitutability of these expressions. Hoffmann's "Fantastic Tales" can be treated like a dream because tales and dreams hold for one another. In this way, the tale "Der Sandmann"—"the Sand-Man," who tears out the eyes of little children, throws them in his sack, and carries them to the moon as fodder for his hook-beaked young—is the equivalent of a dream. The fear expressed here is a substitute for something else, namely, the fear of castration; and this substitution itself becomes "intelligible as soon as we replace the Sand-Man by the dreaded father at whose hands castration is expected" (*S.E.*, 17:232).

Dreams and fairy tales are thus substitutable, just as in a dream and in a fairy tale castration and tearing out eyes are substitutable, just as in the story of the child Nathaniel the father and Coppelius "represent the two opposites into which the father-imago is split by his ambivalence [the child's feelings]; whereas the one threatens to blind him—that is, to castrate him—, the other, the 'good' father, intercedes for his sight" (ibid., p. 232 n). The equivalence of the *modes* of the fantastic (dream and fairy tale) is made possible by reason of the constitutive substitution of the fantasy (tearing out eyes/ punishing). The "uncanny" effect this tale produces comes from an affective material no different from that produced by the return of the repressed in dreams: something that is at once most "familiar" *(heimlich)* to us because most personal, and at the same time seems "strange" *(unheimlich)*, for it has become foreign to us.

One must go perhaps even further. This primordial substitutability belonging to fantasy would explain not only that dreams, tales, myths, and symptoms can be *exchanged* one for another, but that humanity *had to* create works of art just as it has to dream. If substitution is indeed the essence of the fantastic, man had to try to *structure* his fantasies because of the impossibility of an absolutely original return of the repressed. If a *primal* "presentation" is impossible, if a *lived* restitution is impossible, perhaps the only way to rediscover one's childhood, which is behind one, is to create it before oneself, in a work.

This final consequence also marks the return of our initial qualms. They concerned two points: esthetic technique and artistic talent. To what extent have they been removed? As for the first, we might say that the difficulty was circumvented, not resolved. The *effect* on the spectator of the technique of "fore-pleasure" was followed through, but the technique itself continues to be just as impenetrable. Psychoanalysis shows in what way dreams and works of art are *substitutable;* their essential dissymmetry is yet to be understood. It is, in fact, one thing to fantasize at night in dreams. It is something else again to produce in a lasting object—a sculpture, painting, or poem—the single reality that can take the place of this absent original, what we call the impressions of early childhood. It is here that our qualms in regard to the first point are extended to the second one: for if the artist makes a lasting work, it is because he is successful in *structuring* his fantasies outside of himself. In what can this talent possibly consist?

If one has this question in mind, one notes that an essay like "The Moses of Michelangelo" is successful to the extent that this question is bracketed. It is indeed remarkable that the statue is treated as an object isolated from the rest of Michelangelo's work and from the great text of his life. It is compared only to the corresponding biblical text, which is itself isolated from its context (and in addition, in the appendix of 1927, to the Moses of Nicolas de Verdun—that is, to another variant of the archetypal Moses, caught here at the very moment when the storm of passions is being unleashed and not, as in Michelangelo's *Moses*, at the moment when the calm has returned after the storm). Psychoanalysis is *successful*, then, to the extent that it can delimit the structural unity of a "type" (here, the "type" Moses) and can make this unity pass through its diverse textual variants. Freud's scruples begin this side of—or beyond—the case in which the individuality of a variant is to be carried back to the creative genius of an extraordinary personality.

But perhaps it is the question itself that should come under suspicion.

Here, a third argument takes over: if, in the texts we have just examined, Freud does not directly undertake a study of the enigma par excellence, that of artistic *creation*, it will be held that this is because the theme of "talent," of "genius," or of "creation" is not at its basis esthetical but theological. And along with this, that it belongs to a hidden ideology, whose privileged cultural expressions arise from a cultural sphere other than art, one that Freud has indeed marked out *elsewhere*, in his writings on religion. The very idea of a creator, in fact, conserves a religious resonance even in the most rationalistic of minds. It is perhaps in the rationalistic mind that this theological ideology finds its last refuge: is not the creator the father of his works, and thus a *father figure?* As Sarah Kofman writes in *l'Enfance de l'Art*, it is only in a theological conception of art that one can posit "a free

conscious subject, the father of his works as God is of creation"
(p. 20).

Freud's scruples, referred to at the beginning of this essay,
attest to his having admitted, if not in what he *does* at least in
what he *says*, the ideology of genius. Yet the strategic function
of his qualms is revealed when one considers that to shatter the
idol of the artist, the hidden figure of the father, is, in the final
analysis, "to accomplish a murder, that of the artist as genius,
as great man" (Kofman, p. 26). For this reason, the application of psychoanalysis to art encounters the strongest of
resistances. Freud's scruples are held to take this resistance
into account. In order to unmask such resistance in turn, it
would then be enough to "read Freud's texts on art in
accordance with a method of deciphering that he himself has
taught, by distinguishing between what he says and what he
actually does in his discourse" (p. 35). Reading Freud's text
with a suspicious eye would then not risk being arbitrary, but
would conform to the prototype found in Freud's writings on
religion. These texts are held to contain the key to an
auto-critique which, applied to the texts on art, would put an
end to the sort of *auto-censure* that continues to function there,
whether sincerely or as a trick.

In the light of texts such as *The Future of an Illusion, Civilization
and its Discontents*, and *Moses and Monotheism*, the cult of the
genius in art indeed appeared to be cut from the same
instinctual fabric as that of the cult of religious genius. In both
instances, overevaluating the father in early childhood, rival-
ing him, repressing the murder-wish directed toward him, and
finally internalizing his figure, all lead to the same disguises in
sublime figures. The principal difference between the cult of
art and the religion of father is held to lie in the fact that the
artistic phase corresponds to the narcissistic stage, and the
religious phase to that of the cathexis of the libido, to the fixation of the parents—to employ the progressive schema of

Totem and Taboo (which speaks not of the artistic phase but of the animist phase). This parallelism would thus make art "the last bastion of narcissism" (Kofman, p. 35).

This thesis has the advantage of revealing how dangerous it can be to apply psychoanalysis to art. To destroy the idea of genius is to repeat the murder of the father. In the same stroke, "The Moses of Michelangelo" can no longer remain unrelated to *Moses and Monotheism*. By analyzing Michelangelo's statue, does Freud not commit, in regard to the genius of the great sculptor, the same murder that formerly the Hebrews committed in regard to the great prophet? Nor can one leave unrelated the claims of veneration addressed to the "good nature" that resides in creators of art and the attacks against the same idea of the "good nature" of benevolent Providence, when this idea is professed by a religious mind. No, one cannot fail to transfer to the esthetics of genius Freud's own statements in "The Economic Problems of Masochism," in which the terms *Nature, God,* and *Providence* are replaced by *Logos* and *Ananke (S.E.,* 19:168).

This form of argumentation is certainly one of the strongest to be directed against an interpretation that would accept literally the most modest of Freud's statements concerning psychoanalysis's "application" to art. Yet it does not appear to me to entirely resolve the problem.

If, indeed, the ideology of genius blocks out a scientific explanation of artistic talent, one cannot just push it aside in order to account completely for the phenomenon of esthetic creation. I shall say, on the contrary, that by raising the hypothesis of the ideology of genius, Freud exposes the true difficulty, that which concerns the *vicissitude* of instinctual drives in the case of esthetic activity. Now, as soon as the investigation is engaged along this path, one is quick to discover that the qualms expressed in regard to esthetic creation coincide quite precisely with those that Freud ex-

presses elsewhere on the subject of the psychoanalytic treatment of the instinctual vicissitude that he calls "sublimation."

This is what is shown by the text we have held in reserve
until now: *Leonardo da Vinci and a Memory of his Childhood*. One
cannot say of this text what was said above of "The Moses of
Michelangelo," namely, that it avoids the problem of creation
by substituting for it the analysis of a fantasy objectified in
stone, nor that it replaces the problem of creation with that of
the effects produced on the layman. The problem of creation
and creator is instead placed at the center of the work, and the
constellation of fantasies, memories, and creations at the
periphery of the core of instinct of Leonardo the man.

And it is precisely by doing this that Freud comes in contact
with the two enigmas of creation and sublimation, which
resemble one another and form a pair. What in Leonardo has
puzzled most critics? Less his genius than the facts that for him
investigation replaced creation, that his interest was increasingly directed toward science, that even in his artistic activity
he was so peculiarly slow and intermittent—even negligent—
in his work, and finally that he was indifferent to the outcome
of this or that work. Comparing the artist's inhibitions and
Leonardo's distance from sexuality and from his own homosexuality, kept aloof from any possible realization, Freud
confronts the problem which, to my mind, guarantees the
complete coherence of this brief work: the problem of convert-
ing the libido into *sublimated* energy. Sublimation is proposed
here as the third fate of infantile sexual investigation during
the period when repression puts an end to the first attempts at
intellectual independence; alongside neurotic inhibition and
obsession, where thought becomes entirely sexual, there is a
third type, "the rarest and most perfect": here, "the libido
evades the fate of repression by being sublimated from the very
beginning into curiosity and by becoming attached to the
powerful instinct for research as a reinforcement" (*S.E.*,

11:80). It is this capacity to sublimate the greater part of his libido into an instinct for research that makes Leonardo the "prototype of our third type."

If one continues to keep in mind this relation established initially between the peculiar modality of creation in Leonardo and the general problem of sublimation as the fate of instinct, what follows in Freud's work is seen at once to form a coherent whole. The second and third chapters deal with the fantasy that gives the work its title: "a memory of [Leonardo's] childhood," but they include no references to, no mention of, Leonardo's paintings. This point is of the greatest importance for an understanding of Freud's work. For here it is not a question of creation or of sublimation. The entire analysis unfolds within the space of representation and of substitution by which we earlier characterized the *fantastic* as such.

The "memory," as we know, is the famous vulture opening the infant's mouth with its tail. This memory is treated as a construction "after the fact," cast back into childhood. It serves as a link to an entire series of "translations" which reveal nothing other than the capacity for substituting one for another the figures of fantasy, not to mention the dream, mythical, or literary modality of the figures. The "translations" are mutual equivalents in regard to their sense content: the fantasy of passive homosexuality is traded for the image of the maternal breast; the mother is replaced by the vulture in the hieroglyphic writing of the Egyptians; in its turn, the maternal vulture, which according to legend is impregnated by the wind, is traded for the husbandless mother of Leonardo's early childhood. The circle formed by these translations can indeed pass sometimes by way of a private fantasy—which Freud does not hesitate to call the "real content of the memory"; sometimes by way of a mythical symbol—the goddess Mut, image of the phallic mother; and, finally, to close the circle with a fantasy tied to an infantile sexual theory, by the infantile hypothesis of the maternal penis: in all this, Freud does no more than transfer to Leonardo's "case" the most confirmed psychoanalytic theories regarding the laws of fantasy.[8]

In this way, until the *work* has been brought into play, one remains inside a system of pure equivalents, moving from Leonardo's "memory," homosexual dreams, the imaginative structure of the first infantile theories on sex, to the mythical representation of the phallic mother. Something new appears when, beginning with chapter 4, an esthetic object is introduced: the Mona Lisa's *smile*, which is also repeated in the smile of *St. Anne* and in all the "Leonardesque" smiles. In a certain sense—the sense that the theme of the fantastic has revealed up to now—Mona Lisa's smile is interchangeable with the fantasy of the vulture: "it was his mother who possessed the mysterious smile—the smile that he had lost and that had fascinated him so much when he found it again in the Florentine lady" (*S.E.*, 11:111). In *this* sense, it is his mother's smile, the memory of which was awakened by the Florentine lady, that is painted on the canvas; it is this smile which, at the period when the *St. Anne* was painted, "drove him at once to create a glorification of motherhood, and to give back to his mother the smile he had found in the noble lady" (p. 112). Thus Freud can say that "The picture contains the synthesis of the history of his childhood: its details are to be explained by reference to the most personal impressions in Leonardo's life" (p. 112).

Such is the interpretation within the limits of Freud's theory of fantasy, marked by the dual trait of respresentability and of substitutability. The equivalence of the painted smile and the fantasy of the vulture seems to be perfect: the "same" infantile

---

8. On two occasions, Freud even makes Leonardo's unconscious speak through the psychoanalytic translation: "That was a time when my fond curiosity was directed to my mother and when I still believed she had a genital organ like my own" (*S.E.*, 11:98). And: "through this erotic relation with my mother . . . I became a homosexual" (p. 106).

impression engenders both. Leonardo "strove to reproduce the smile with his brush, giving it to all his pictures." (p. 117).

But there follows immediately a slight adjustment that destroys the equivalence: "It is possible that in these figures Leonardo has denied *[verleugnet]* the unhappiness of his erotic life and has triumphed over it in his art *[und Künstlerisch überwunden]*, by representing the wishes of the boy, infatuated with his mother, as fulfilled in this blissful union of the male and the female natures" (pp. 117-18). These words alone— *denied* and *triumphed over*—express, *in regard to* the work itself, the enigma of sublimation *in* the dynamics of instinctual drives. *In regard to* the work, sublimation signifies that the fantasy and the painting are not interchangeable: one can go from the work to the fantasy; one cannot find the work in the fantasy. What is expressed in economic terms as "the libido's abandoning its immediate goal in favor of other non-sexual goals, ultimately more elevated in the minds of men" (chap. 1), this is expressed in objective terms as the elevation of the fantasy to a work.

Transposing the famous saying *wo es war, soll ich werden*— "where there was *id*, there must be *ego*"—one is tempted to say, where there was the fantasy of the vulture, there must come to be the mother's smile as a pictorial work. The enigma of the Mona Lisa's smile is not that of the fantasy of the vulture. For the painted smile does not repeat any real memory, neither that of the lost mother nor that of the Florentine lady whose encounter triggered the regression to the childhood memory and kindled the new erotic flare-up, more powerful than his inhibitions. The celebrated smile—the Leonardesque smile— is a figurative innovation in relation to any repetition of fantasies. The work of art is not limited to exhibiting the object of a wish; for the kisses of the first mother, the lost mother, are themselves lost insofar as they are real memories; the fantasy is always a substitute for something absent that is signified, its sole presence is that created by the painter; the true smile, which will be sought in vain, is not behind in some actual event that could be relived, it is in front of us, on the painted canvas.[9]

The entire theoretical enigma of substitution is concentrated here in the passage from a single "mental derivative"—the fantasy—to a work which from this moment on exists in the cultural bank. Leonardo's brush does not re-create the memory of his mother, but creates it as a work of art, by creating *the* smile as seen by Leonardo.

It is no longer possible to set in opposition here what Freud *does* and what he *says*. He makes an affective difficulty of interpretation coincide with a theoretical difficulty of metapsychology. It was, in fact, the underlying difficulty in the previous analysis as well. Why were *Oedipus Rex* and *Hamlet*, as poems, capable of impressing the seal of universality on a dream, even on a "typical" one? Why, if not for the reason that dreams, the typical and sterile products of our nights, have already been *"denied"* and *"overcome"* in a lasting creation of our days? Sublimation has thus been anticipated in the universalizing function of the esthetic model of dreams. The meaning of dreams is not only less hidden here, and for this reason more readable, but is produced as meaning in a space other than the space of fantasy, that is, in the cultural space.

That sublimation itself continued to be a great enigma to Freud is abundantly confirmed by his continuing allusions to this problem. The first of the *Three Essays on Sexuality* characterizes sublimation by the deviation of the libido's goal rather

9. On this point, I have nothing to change in the analysis I proposed in *Freud and Philosophy:* "The Gioconda's smile undoubtedly takes us back to the childhood memory of Leonardo da Vinci, but this memory only exists as a symbolizable absence that lies deep beneath Mona Lisa's smile. Lost like a memory, the mother's smile is an empty place within reality; it is the point where all real traces become lost, where the abolished confines one to fantasy. It is not therefore a thing that is better known and that would explain the riddle of the work of art; it is an intended absence which, far from dissipating the initial riddle, increases it" (pp. 173–74).

than by the substitution of the object. Along the way he attaches to it the notion of the bonus of seduction and of fore-pleasure, whose use in esthetics we saw earlier. But he then admits in the same essay: "But we must end with a confession that very little is as yet known with certainty of these pathways, though they certainly exist and can probably be traversed in both directions" (*S.E.*, 7:206). In the last essay, which compares sublimation to repression, Freud says expressly that these are processes "of which the inner causes are quite unknown to us" (p. 239). In his essay "On Narcissism" sublimation is contrasted with rather than compared to idealization.

The more Freud distinguishes sublimation from other mechanisms, particularly from repression and even from reaction-formation, the more its own mechanism lies unexplained: it is a displacement of energy but not a repression of it; it indeed appears to be related to an aptitude with which the artist is particularly gifted. At the time of *The Ego and the Id*, the emphasis is placed on the conversion of object-libido into narcissistic libido and on desexualization; such desexualization, he adds, is "a kind of sublimation, therefore. Indeed, the question arises, and deserves careful consideration, whether this is not the universal road to sublimation, whether all sublimation does not take place through the mediation of the ego, which begins by changing sexual object-libido into narcissistic libido and then, perhaps, goes on to give it another aim" (*S.E.*, 19:30). As we see, sublimation is as much the heading of a problem as the name of a solution.

Faced with such difficulties, one understands that Freud must be taken *literally* precisely when he says, in his *Leonardo*: "Since artistic talent and capacity are intimately connected with sublimation we must admit that the nature of the artistic function is also inaccessible to us along psycho-analytic lines" (*S.E.*, 11:136).

But by recognizing that psychoanalysis has real limits, the

philosopher who reflects and meditates on them discovers at the same time what such limits mean for a theory that unceasingly advances on the unknown: these limits are not fixed boundaries; they are as mobile as the investigation itself and, in this sense, are indefinitely surmountable.

REFERENCES

Freud, Sigmund. *Standard Edition of the Complete Psychological Works.* London: Hogarth, 1953–66.
"Extracts from the Fliess Papers," vol. 1
The Interpretation of Dreams, vols. 4, 5
Three Essays on Sexuality, vol. 7
Jokes and their Relation to the Unconscious, vol. 8
"Creative Writers and Day-dreaming," vol. 9
Leonardo da Vinci and a Memory of his Childhood, vol. 11
Totem and Taboo, vol. 13
"The Moses of Michelangelo," vol. 13
"The Unconscious," vol. 14
"The 'Uncanny,' " vol. 17
"The Economic Problem of Masochism," vol. 19
The Future of an Illusion, vol. 21
Civilization and its Discontents, vol. 21
Moses and Monotheism, vol. 23
Freud, Sigmund. *An Autobiographical Study.* Translated by James Strachey. New York: Norton, 1952.
Kofman, Sarah. *l'Enfance de l'Art.* Paris: Payot, 1970.
Ricoeur, Paul. *Freud and Philosophy.* Translated by Denis Savage. New Haven: Yale University Press, 1970.

2

Observations on Psychoanalysis and Modern Literature*

Erich Heller

In the history of thought it occurs again and again that a privileged mind turns a long-nurtured suspicion into a system and puts it to the good, or not so good, uses of teachers and learners. When this happens, we say that it has been in the air for a long time. This is so in the case of psychoanalysis, and whatever its future fate, its historical importance is beyond doubt. For it is impossible not to come into contact with it or to avoid the collision, even if one merely wanted to say to it that it has no business being there. A theory owes this kind of inescapability to its long maturation in the womb of Time. It is born and casts its spell upon a world that seems to have been prepared for quite a while to receive it. Pallas Athene, it is said, sprang from her father's head in full armor. But surely, before this birth took place Zeus must have spent many a day pondering Athenian thoughts and must have done so in the Athenian dialect; and our world had awaited Freud long before it heard his name.

This is why psychoanalysis appears to be more than merely one among many possible theories about the psyche; rather, it comes close to being the systematic consciousness that a certain epoch has of the nature and character of its soul.

* Erich Heller's essay, written for this volume, also appeared in the quarterly *Salmagundi*, 10th anniversary issue (Fall, 1975).

Therefore it would be an endless enterprise to speak of Freud's influence on modern literature; and literature, whatever else it may be, is also the esthetic form assumed by the self-awareness of an age. If a writer today speaks of fathers or sons, of mothers or dreams, of lovers or rivals, of accidents that determine destinies or destinies rooted in character, of the will to live or the longing for death—and what else is it that poets and writers talk about?—how can he remain untouched by Freudian thoughts even if he has never read a line by Freud? And the more he were to try to extinguish or "repress" this "influence," the more he would become its victim. Could a post-Freudian poet say what Goethe's Egmont says: "As if whipped on by invisible demons, the sun-born horses of Time rush along with the fragile chariot of our destiny, and nothing is left to us but intrepidly to hold fast to the reins and keep the wheels from pushing against a wall of rock or driving into an abyss" (*Egmont*, 2:2)—could a contemporary writer put such words into the mouth of his hero without suspecting that he has learned it from Freud?—that the invisible demons with their whip are really the unconscious, the id, and the rather helpless charioteer, the ego with its good intentions?

From Goethe, Novalis, the German arch-Romantic, and Kleist, the one and only naturally tragic poet of German literature (even if Goethe once cursed him as *"Unnatur"*— *"Diese verdammte Unnatur,"* he said), and certainly from the literature we have uppermost in mind when speaking of the later nineteenth century—from Stendhal, Flaubert, and de Maupassant, from Tolstoi and Dostoievski—there is a much shorter way to Freud than the maps of literary history usually show; and the subsequent literature is altogether domiciled in a country the cartographer of which is Freud. It may not be the most pertinent of questions to ask whether Hofmannsthal, Schnitzler, Broch, Musil, Kafka, Rilke, Hermann Hesse, or Thomas Mann have been "influenced" by Freud, or whether Joyce or Virginia Woolf, Hemingway or Faulkner have "learned" from him; for the question—to which the answer may be in some cases yes and more frequently no—is almost as irrelevant as it would be to ask whether the first builders of aircraft were inspired by Newton. Airplanes fly in Newtonian space, trusting, as it were, in the validity of the law of gravity. What, then, are the qualities of the sphere of the psyche traversed by modern literature?

Out of its multitudinous characteristics I wish to select two from the writings of Thomas Mann. The first bears upon the problem of man's responsibility for his decisions and actions— that is, the problem of morality itself. A masterpiece among novellas, *Death in Venice*, supplies our first example. We remember the episode (in the third section of the story) that is decisive in the development of the plot, when Gustav von Aschenbach for the last time tries to take the moral initiative in the encounter with his destiny. He wants to escape from the sickly oppression—from the Venetian air, heavy and sultry with the sirocco, where the deadly epidemic would soon luxuriate, but also from his growing passion for the beautiful boy Tadzio. He determines to leave and orders his luggage to be taken to the railway station on the hotel's early-morning motor boat, whereas he himself, believing that there is enough time for an unrushed breakfast and, without acknowledging this to himself, perhaps for a last silent encounter with Tadzio, chooses to take a later public steamship. But when he arrives at the station, his luggage has gone off on a wrong train. This accident makes his moral determination collapse. He decides to wait for his trunk in Venice, returns to his Lido hotel and to his erotic enchantment. He is ready now for the approaching disease and for death.

Fate and accident are ancient allies; yet only in the Freudian era could *this* accident have been woven in this manner into the texture of destiny. For as Thomas Mann tells the story, the accident is not, as any similar event in Greek tragedy would be, a weapon in the hands of a divine antagonist with whom the hero's will is interlocked in combat, and not a cunning maneuver of that friend or foe called Fate. It is rather the revelation of Aschenbach's true will that gives the lie to his declared intention to depart. If Aschenbach is clearly innocent of the mistake made in the dispatching of his luggage, he is innocent only after the canon of traditional moral judgments. According to the new dispensation he is responsible; and in his soul he knows this, or comes to know it, as he ecstatically welcomes that travel mishap as if it were the gift of freedom itself. "Aschenbach," we read, "found it hard to let his face assume the expression that the news of the mishap required, for he was almost convulsed with reckless delight, an unbelievable joy."

The basic idea of Thomas Mann's novel *The Magic Mountain* can be stated almost in one sentence: Hans Castorp, a seemingly "well-adjusted" young shipbuilding engineer from Hamburg, has planned a visit of three weeks in a Swiss sanatorium for tubercular diseases where his cousin is a patient, but remains there for seven years. Certainly, he becomes ill himself, but his physical symptoms are by no means serious. What then is the *real* reason for his tarrying? It is his hidden wish, a secret perhaps to himself, to await the return of Clavdia Chauchat. He has fallen in love with the Russian woman, and she, as she leaves, promises that she will return: and Hans Castorp waits seven years. His illness is merely a pretext for his waiting. Against all "humanistic" reasonableness and moral principles, his *true* will has asserted itself. And Thomas Mann began to read Freud only *after* he had written *The Magic Mountain*. Voilà, the Zeitgeist!

Both *Death in Venice* and *The Magic Mountain* would be unthinkable were it not for the Romantic fascination with the alliance between love and sickness and death; and this is almost as much as to say: unthinkable without depth psychology. These works are situated in a territory of the psyche the

ethics of which are radically different from those of the
Enlightenment (to name only one of the preceding epochs). It
is strange that the strongest hostile response evoked by Freud's
teaching was, at least to begin with, moral indignation. Freud,
it was held, undermined morality and catastrophically nar-
rowed the domain in which ethical laws could be applied
unquestioningly. A profounder criticism would have been to
show that, on the contrary, he extended a person's responsibility so immeasurably that it became in practice all but
unworkable.

The rationalistic doctrine of morality, which until the
Romantic period had dominated the moral philosophy of
Western civilization, saw the moral person triumph or suc-
cumb in a *conscious* struggle with forces which, no matter
whether they were called "nature" or "instinct" or "inclination," were the simple antagonists of the ethically wakeful
human being. In Freud's doctrine, deeply indebted to the
Romantic sensibility, the moral conflict becomes total warfare.
It is waged even in places where once upon a time the warrior
sought and found relaxation from the strains of morality: in
sleep, in dreams, in fantasies, in innocently involuntary action.
Let anyone say now: "I have only dreamt this," or "I did not
intend to say this; it was a mere slip of the tongue," or "I was
determined to do what I promised, but then I forgot":
instantly he will be persuaded that he dreamt what he dreamt,
said what he said, forgot what he forgot, because he was
prompted by his deepest and truest will. While the moralist of
the rational Enlightenment proved himself or failed in what
he consciously *willed* or *did,* the Romantic and Freudian
morality is once again concerned with the innermost character
of a person, with his *being.* Once again; for there was a time,
long ago, when a prophet struck fear and terror—albeit by
speaking in a different idiom—into the minds of the Pharisees
by putting the goodness of the hidden soul or the rebirth of the

whole man ethically above righteous observance of the law by the publicly displayed good will. This was the essence of the moral revolution of Christianity.

As psychoanalysis, with all its variations and eclectic modifications, is a dominant part of the epoch's consciousness, it has a share in its calamity. This manifests itself—speaking, as would seem appropriate, in medical terms—in the vast superiority of presumed diagnostic insights over therapeutic possibilities. Has there ever been a doctor who has diagnosed as many pathological irritations as Freud? The psyche is to him an inexhaustible reservoir of abnormalities, precariously dammed in by the most delicate concept of health. All pleasures and all oppressions of the soul, all sins and all virtues, restlessness of the heart as well as the great constancy of love, fear of evil as well as faith in God—all these may in the twinkling of the diagnostic eye degenerate into signs of psychic imbalance. But what is the health of the soul? Compared to the resourcefulness and ingenuity of the diagnosis, the only answer that can be given within the limits of psychology is primitive, pedestrian, and simple-minded: the ability to control the controllable conditions of existence and the adjustment to the unalterable. But who has drawn the frontier between the controllable and the unalterable? Where exactly does it run? Is it fixed by God, this fabrication of the father-bound neurotic psyche? Or by nature who has created the boy after the image of Oedipus and then handed him over to the healing practices of psychological *ratio?* Or by society or the state? By *which* society and *which* state? By that Victorian society whose numerous pathological symptoms have called forth psychoanalysis? Or by the enlightened, generously liberal, thoroughly "demythologized" society that on both sides of the Atlantic sends swarms of patients into the consulting rooms of psychologists? Or by the tyrannical state that prohibits their activities?

The questions are endless and unanswerable. For it is true

to say that if there were an answer, there would be no
psychoanalysis. It would not have been invented had it not
been for the disappearance from our beliefs of any certainty
concerning the nature of human being. Thus we have become
the incurable patients of our all but nihilistic skepticism,
indulging a conception of the soul that stipulates more, many
more, psychic possibilities than can be contained in one
existence. Whichever possibilities we choose, we miss out on
the others—and distractedly feel our loss without being able
ethically to justify it. Inevitably foregoing uncounted possibilities, we experience this as the betrayal of a vaguely conceived
"fullness of life." For our beliefs do not acknowledge any
reason to sacrifice possibilities in order to gain our reality—a
reality that for us has assumed the character of the arbitrary
and the indefinable. Thus we are haunted by as many dead
possibilities as there is room for in the wide region of
frustrations. It is the accomplished hypochondria of unbelief.

Paradoxically enough, Freud himself, over long stretches of
his enterprise, was securely at home in that rationalistic
Enlightenment faith whose increasing instability was the
historical occasion of his doctrine, just as the doctrine in its
turn added to the disturbance. But because he himself was
hardly affected by it, he had no ear for the question his own
theory raised, and certainly did not have the *philosophical*
genius to meet it. With astonishing naïveté he examined the
"how" of psychic conditions, as if such labors could yield clear
answers to the "what" of psychic phenomena, of their meaning
and their possible relatedness to the possibly true nature of
being. Thus he believed, for instance, that primeval murderers
of their fathers created from the agony of their guilt a
godfather to be worshipped—a theory which, of course,
presupposes that those savage creatures in all their savagery
possessed a conscience and the psychic disposition to believe in
God. Yet Freud did not ask to what end human beings should
have the ability to feel guilty or the capacity for religious

beliefs, but took for granted that the conscience and the faith of his savages corresponded to nothing real in the world and fed on sheer illusions; and his readers, just as he himself did, looked upon certain *contents* of guilt and faith understandably as being antiquated, without paying attention to the *form* and quality of these psychic dispositions. But are those dispositions not exceedingly curious if they have no correlative whatever in the order of reality? Of course, Freud would rightly have said that this was not a psychological question, but a metaphysical or ontological one. True. But to doubt the very validity of such questions, quite apart from the inability to answer them, is the main psychological characteristic of the epoch that has produced psychoanalysis as its representative psychology.

One of its most important tenets is the theory of repression. From the beginning of his history man has suffered from the compulsion to "repress," and only because he "represses" has he a history, for historical epochs or cultures differ one from the other by the changing molds in which they cast some human possibilities at the expense of others. This is why the ancient Greeks were, despite Pythagoras and the Pythagoreans, not rich in great natural scientists, but in artistic accomplishments unsurpassed by any other age; or why we have the most self-assured and effective technology, but arts that are exceedingly tentative, uncertain, restless, and experimental; or why creations of nature have been, ever since the discovery of Nature, the great comfort and pleasure of the Romantic sensibility: because this tree or that range of mountains appears to be the sum total, without loss or sacrifice, of *all* its potentialities, and therefore never hurts our esthetic sense by insinuating to us that it might have done much better had it only chosen another career. For one of the things that set man apart from all other beings is that the sum of his potentialities by far exceeds the measure of their realizability in one human life or even in one historical epoch. Man has been given language (in the sense of all his means of expression) so that he can say what he has not chosen to be silent about. He is such an eloquent creature because he is unspeakably secretive. This is the natural-historical aspect of human transcendence, the psychological side of his "existential problem."

Human existence is choice, resignation, sacrifice—and, indeed, neurotic repression if a man has to make his inescapable choices and sacrifices under the dim enforcement of social norms he no longer believes in, instead of basing his decisions upon the belief in the greater virtue of what he has chosen, no matter whether he does so consciously or unconsciously, from lucid insight or from faithful, unreflective obedience. If he no longer feels that there is any compelling reason why he should forego this in order to achieve that, if his existence is not illuminated by any shimmer of its transcendence, then his rejected potentialities (or, for that matter, injuries sustained by the child in his religiously or ethically "agnostic" society) grow into neuroses in the darkness of the unconscious. And psychoanalysis shares with existential philosophy the tragic fate that, although it is, of course, founded upon the awareness of the universal human need to choose, to select, and to sacrifice, it is at the same time, like most other creations of the age, deprived of the means to transcend this distressing human condition.

From this follows the "scientific" intention of psychoanalysis to disregard any hierarchy that religion or metaphysics or ethics or tradition has set up concerning the activities of consciousness. It may well be true to say that this has been the first such attempt in the history of man's efforts to know himself. There is for psychoanalysis no preestablished order of the psyche: it is impossible to discern, at least initially, what is important to it and what is unimportant. It is a theory that lets itself in with chaos. If there is to be any order, it has to be created—somewhat in keeping with the aperçu of that arch-Romantic Novalis (in his celebrated fragment of 1799, "Christendom or Europe") that only anarchy will once again beget a true spiritual order: "Religion will rise from the chaos of destruction as the glorious founder of a new world." [1]

Psychoanalysis—like the sensibility of romanticism (as opposed to that of classicism)—is imbued with the suspicion that everything, every tatter of a dream, every scrap of memory, every seemingly arbitrary association our thinking makes between this and that, may be of hitherto unsuspected significance within the economy of the soul, just as Marcel (in the first volume of Proust's vast novel *À la recherche du temps perdu*) receives those sudden messages of a great and hidden truth, those unpredictable intimations of eternity, from a stone the surface of which reflected the sunlight, or from the clanging of a bell, or from the smell of fallen leaves—"a confused mass of different images, under which must have perished long ago the reality"—the absolute reality he was seeking. Nietzsche's great and truly dreadful experiment consisted in his assuming that the history of the Western mind was nothing but a conspiracy to conceal the truth; and where such concealment is looked upon as the rule, the suspicion is bound to arise that, vice versa, anything—literally anything—may unexpectedly "conduct" the mind toward a tremendous illumination. It is precisely this that distinguishes modern literature from, above all, the myth-bound poetry of ancient Greece. And what Hofmannsthal said, in his poem "Lebenslied," of the "heir" of this long process of disinheritance, is as true of psychoanalysis as it is of the artist of the psychoanalytical age:

> Ihm bietet jede Stelle
> Geheimnisvoll die Schwelle—

meaning that he who is without a home in an ordered world will entrust himself to any current of chance to take him

1. Novalis, *Fragmente*, ed. Ernst Kamnitzer (Dresden: Wolfgang Yess Verlag, 1929), p. 738.

anywhere, for anywhere may be the threshold of the mystery.

Proust's great novelistic oeuvre, the attempt to catch hold of a withdrawing world by means of an exquisitely woven net of memories; James Joyce's *Ulysses*, this monster work of genius that turns the experience of one day into a kind of lyrical-epical encyclopedia; Hermann Broch's time-consuming record of Virgil's dying; not to mention the many minor "stream of consciousness" novels—all these are the literary products of an epoch whose soul has been analyzed by Sigmund Freud. And whatever will remain of this literature will bear the imprint of a consciousness that Freud has helped to become conscious of itself—and thus, given the nature of consciousness, has helped to come into being. But can a consciousness that is so thoroughly conscious of itself ever achieve that *"geprägte Form,"* as Goethe called it in *"Urworte-Orphisch,"* the oneness of deliberate form and "naïve" spontaneity that has always been the hallmark of great art?

Speaking of Freud and modern literature, we cannot help concerning ourselves with the unusual, and in all probability critical, situation of literature in an age that is constantly in search of an acceptable theory of its soul. For the relationship of art to that self-understanding of the soul which culminates in Freud is by no means free of conflicts, and these tensions have been in the making ever since the truth about man has been sought not in myth or religion but in psychology. Psychology—the psychology, for instance, that dominates the novel of the nineteenth century—is the science of disillusionment. Its climate is, as some of the Romantics believed, unfavorable to poetry; and in a serious sense it is true to say that the history of the psychological novel is the progressive dissolution of what traditionally has been regarded as poetic. Novalis, who wrote that psychology is one of the "ghosts" that have "usurped the place in the sanctuary where the monuments of gods should be," knew what he did when he countered the Romantic enthusiasm for Goethe's *Wilhelm*

Meister, indeed his own fascination with that novel, by calling it a "Candide aimed at poetry," a satire of the poetic mode.[2]

Goethe, in his turn, accused Kleist, this *Ur*-patient and *Ur*-practitioner of depth analysis, of aiming at the confusion of feelings. What he meant by this was very likely the war that Kleist's imagination, in love with the heroic and the mythic, fought with his analytical intelligence; and this intelligence was at the same time in unrelenting pursuit of the psychological truth. It is a feud that reverberates throughout Kleist's dramatic verse and prose. Indeed, the source of the particular fascination wielded by his dramas and stories is the clash, and at times the unquiet marriage, between poetry and neurosis. Goethe was bound to abhor this poet as intensely as Kafka admired him. For Goethe believed—at least at times—that poetry prospered only when it was left to grow and mature in the unconscious. He said so to Schiller in a letter of April 6, 1801, and added that poetry presupposes in those who make it "a certain good-natured and even simple-minded love for the real which is the hiding-place of truth."

Unconscious, good-natured, simple-minded, trusting that the hidden truth may, after all, reveal itself to the naïve mind in the phenomenal world—if one were to define Kleist's genius, indeed the spirit of modern literature, by means of its perfect opposite, this would be its negative definition. Should it ever happen that a history of modern literature is written in honor of Sigmund Freud—by a literary historian who also possesses a thorough knowledge of psychoanalysis without having become intellectually enslaved by it—it might begin with Goethe's highly conscious praise of the unconscious; contemplate afterwards the Kleistean tension between mythology and psychology, which is at the same time so characteristic of a whole literary epoch; and then arrive at the writings of Nietzsche, that astonishing prompter of psychoanalysis, "the

2. Ibid., pp. 381, 633.

first psychologist of Europe," as, not very modestly, he called himself (and Freud himself all but acknowledged his claim)— Nietzsche, who at the same time never tired of pointing to the perils of the mind's psychological pursuit of itself, and believed he knew that there was a kind of knowledge that may become "a handsome instrument for perdition." [3] Such an essay in literary history might conclude with Kafka's dictum from "Reflections on Sin, Suffering, Hope, and the True Way": "Never again psychology!"

In honor of Sigmund Freud? Would it not, rather, be a polemical performance? No. For is the stance of the polemicist appropriate to the inevitable? Our imaginary historian of literature would show that there is a compelling logical development from German Romanticism, the fountainhead of so many currents in modern literature, to the works of Sigmund Freud. How is this?—the medical sobriety of the founder of psychoanalysis brought into the vicinity of a literary-philosophical movement that is reputed to have fostered every conceivable extravagance of the fancy? Still, the connection exists; and it is a mistaken belief, hardly more than a facile superstition, that the early German Romantics were bent simply on discrediting realistic wakefulness in order to rescue the dreamily poetic, or on fortifying the domain of the imagination against the encroachments of the real.

True, the poet in Novalis was sometimes outraged by the prosaic realism of Goethe's *Wilhelm Meister*. On these occasions he would say of it that it elevated "the economic nature of man" to the rank of his "only true nature" (and he might have said: the nature of man insofar as it is accessible to psychology); or that it was "a piece of poetic machinery to deal with recalcitrant material"; or that with this novel he made his final bid for quasi-bourgeois respectability: "The Pilgrim's Progress toward a knighthood." But in a different mood he

3. *Gesammelte Werke* (Munich: Musarion Verlag, 1922), 6:48.

called it a supreme masterpiece, "the novel *par excellence*," and its author "the true vicar of the poetic spirit on earth." [4] It is clear that even Novalis, the true poet in the first group of German Romantics, played his part in the strategy of Romantic irony, an attitude of mind that would surely be useless in any ferocious defense of the imagination against the attacks of rationality. No, Romantic irony is a play played around a center of great seriousness. Its ambition is to save the authentic life of the imagination from the wreckage of illusions. Just as lifeboat instruction is given on luxurious ocean liners, so Romantic irony aims at teaching the spirit of poetry how to keep afloat in the approaching floods of what Goethe named the Prosaic Age: the Age of Analysis.

Friedrich Schlegel, the Grand Intellectual Master of the early Romantics, demanded that poetry should be practiced like a science, while every science should become a new kind of poetry. This was Schlegel's outré manner of expressing what Schiller, in his celebrated essay "On Spontaneous and Reflective Poetry," hoped for: that at the highest point of consciousness man would acquire a new and higher "naïveté." Novalis said even more: "Those who uncritically believe in their health make the same mistake as those who uncritically regard themselves as sick: both are diseased"—because, one assumes, of their want of critical alertness; and still more, that certain kinds of physical sickness are best treated through treating the psyche, because the soul has the same influence upon the body that the body has upon the soul. If these sayings were offered as utterances of Freud's, the attribution would not meet with much incredulity. And the following *is* all but said by Freud, although it was said by Novalis too: "All that is involuntary must come under the control of the conscious will." [5] This means the same as "*Ego* shall be where *Id* was."

4. Novalis, *Fragmente*, pp. 632–33, 656, 652.
5. Ibid., p. 383.

As one reads what Freud says of the relationship between "I" and "It," of the wounds which the struggles between the two inflict upon the soul, and how the soul may regain its lost integrity through the enhanced consciousness of itself, it is impossible not to relate this great psychological utopia to the vision of a future paradise with which Kleist ends his meditations "On the Marionette Theatre"—or rather, on the neurotic derangement, the false self-consciousness, of the inhibited psyche; and even though the Eden of original innocence and unselfconscious grace is shut for ever, we must, Kleist writes, "embark on the journey around the world in order to find out whether we may not be received through a back door." In the future *perfection of consciousness*, we may recover what we lost in the Fall; we shall have to "eat of the Tree of Knowledge again to fall back into the state of innocence."

Schiller, in that essay on "Spontaneous and Reflective Poetry," means something similar, if not the same, when he speaks of our gaining a new and purified spontaneity through the infinite increase of our reflective power. And what else is it that the philosopher of Romantic pessimism, Schopenhauer, has in mind when he, intimately knowing the terror of the *Id*, the dark impulses of the will, glorifies in his magnum opus, *The World as Will and Idea*, the freedom that the *Ego* may attain through the understanding of that *Id* and itself? And finally Freud and Nietzsche: even if the mountain tops of the prophet Zarathustra seem worlds apart from the consulting room of the analyst, they are nonetheless neighbors, and not only in the sequence of time. For one of Nietzsche's two divinities is Dionysus, the god of the intoxicated will to live—but the other is Apollo, the god who possesses the power of clear articulation and disciplined insight. Nietzsche, too, longed for the ultimate rule of Apollo—not *over* Dionysus but *together with him* in an utopian oneness of mind and will, intellect and impulse.

Yet Nietzsche and Freud are neighbors above all by

virtue—virtue? well, sometimes it seems a necessity imposed by history—by virtue of the determination with which they pursued the truths of psychology, a psychological radicalism intolerant of any gods that were not more than the illusory comforters of sick souls. But if the unimaginable day ever comes when men, beyond sickness and illusion, live in the integrity of being, then the spirits of Freud and Nietzsche may give their assent to Kafka's resolve, unrealizable in his time: "Never again psychology!"

3

Liberation and Self-Destruction in the Creative Process*

HELM STIERLIN

Liberation is primarily a political and social concept. As such, it evokes images of shackles thrown away, of resurging life and hope, of release from oppression and exploitation, of revolution. But liberation is also a psychological and relational concept. As such, it reveals vicissitudes of personal growth, of individuation, yet also of psychological exploitation and self-destruction. In the following essay I want to examine some of these vicissitudes and, for this purpose, shall begin with that phase in life which, I believe, fatefully shapes all our later efforts at liberation—early childhood.

The Interweaving of Liberative and Creative Forces in the Child

To do so, let me focus on a phenomenon which the late D. W. Winnicott, the noted British analyst and pediatrician, described. I have in mind what Winnicott (1953) called *transitional objects*. These transitional objects, according to Winnicott, figure centrally in a child's first separation from his mother. Typically, they are objects such as blankets, dolls, or

* This paper was presented at the Symposium on Literature and Psychology, University of Michigan Center for Coordination of Ancient and Modern Studies, Ann Arbor, Michigan, Nov. 28–Dec. 1, 1973. Parts of it have been incorporated into a forthcoming study, "Hitler: A Family Perspective."

teddy bears, which, to the child, come to embody mother's attributes, particularly her warmth and protective presence. These objects now allow the child to hang onto his mother in a concrete way, but also to control and manipulate her according to his needs. We can say he has now the best of two worlds. He carries his mother with him, as it were, yet also can get rid of her when he wishes: he has autonomy, yet can also bask in dependence. In this way, the child makes a decisive liberative move.

At the same time—and this is now important—the child achieves a creative feat. For he reconciles what seems irreconcilable—namely, autonomy and dependence. That, however —the reconciliation of the seemingly irreconcilable in a new and usually more intricate pattern (be this behavioral, relational, or esthetic)—is, I believe, the essence of the creative process. Thus, by recruiting transitional objects, the child embarks on a creative as well as liberative venture.

However, as he matures, the child reaches a critical threshold at which his creativity and liberation may surge as well as falter. This threshold arrives when he begins to move into the world of words and symbols, when he begins to appropriate his culture through fairy tales, nursery rhymes, and similar elements. To understand what this involves, we must turn to some observations of Winnicott's—those pertaining to what he variously called the area of cultural activity, of play, or of artistic illusion (Winnicott, 1967). H. Lincke (1973), a Swiss psychoanalyst, has also written on this subject.

Winnicott located this area between the areas of "subjective experience," as obtaining in dreams and fantasies, and "objective experience," as shaped by societal institutions and language (which Hegel, in 1810, called the realm of the "objective spirit"). Therefore, Winnicott spoke here also of the "intermediate area." Within this intermediate area, transitional objects increasingly lose their concreteness—in other words, teddy bears become pictures of teddy bears, and pictures of teddy bears become words or symbols representing teddy bears. These words and symbols can still powerfully evoke the mother's warmth and presence, as well as innumerable other things, yet now allow even more leeway for manipulation and reconciliation than do concrete teddy bears and blankets.

In introducing this intermediate area, Winnicott brought into view some of the dilemmas we must face when we want to liberate ourselves and also want to be—or remain—creative.

First, he made understandable why human beings, as children, almost cannot *not* be creative. For all children are plunged head on into this intermediate area, as it were. While their world still glows with pristine brilliance, and emotional currents still break forth easily, they must, willy-nilly, create meaning by linking new images, new things, and new words (even though, or because, they often cannot yet distinguish among the three). Hence the frequent originality of their utterances, hence the freshness of their paintings and drawings, hence the inventiveness of their play, hence their charm.

But, as they grow older—and this, too, appears to follow from Winnicott's observations—children seem to find it ever more difficult to operate creatively in the intermediate area: they are now pulled either into the area of purely subjective experience—that of mere dreams or fantasies—or into that of mere objective experience—the area of conformity to traditional patterns of thought and action. In either case, they lose their creative edge.

To be sure, not a few people dispute the above and consider dreaming and fantasizing to be creative activities. For example, they hold that in dreaming we all turn into creative visionaries and playwrights, as we conjure images resplendent with meaning, plot bold dramas, connect the seemingly unconnectable, speak the unspeakable, reveal whilst we conceal, and display an ingenuity which later makes us and our analysts marvel.

Yet such creativity of dreamers, we know, tends to wither quickly under the waking life's glare. For only rarely does the creative momentum of dreams carry over into immediate wakeful productivity, as it did for Kekulé when he found the formula of the benzene ring in 1865. (This applies also to states of altered consciousness—such as those caused by LSD, marijuana, or peyote—which resemble dream states and which, like dreams, seem to unleash creative forces. For here, also, visions emerge out of the soul's archaic layers, colors intensify, new links and meanings appear, and horizons expand. Yet here, too, the creative surge—if we can call it that—tends to falter soon and ordinarily does not produce lasting achievement. On the contrary, many drug users, huddling together ever more passively, also seem increasingly to lose their zest for life.)

Thus, while dreams might have the emotional charge and imaginative power of true art, they seem too far removed from the realm of durable, objective experiences—namely, the realm of enduringly shared words, symbols, and experiential structures—to deserve the name of creative achievements.

Yet those human productions which adhere too much to such objective experience—that is, fit in too closely with established modes of thought and perception—do not impress us as creative, as they remain stuck in well-worn tracks. Creative activity, it follows, remains precariously lodged in Winnicott's intermediate area, combining in a unique mixture that which is private *and* public, real *and* illusionary, subjective *and* objective; and this mixture, evidently, is hard to achieve.

The Artist's Task of Reconciliation

Still, certain individuals do achieve it, and they, the truly creative artists, are thus the proper subjects for any deeper examination of the creative process. Let me, then, turn to them. These artists—and here I want to focus chiefly on creative writers—refuse to be dislodged from the intermediate realm, even while they grow older, as they neither merely dream nor merely follow established tracks. How do they do it?

They do it, first of all, by remaining childlike in important respects. Like children, artists seem to retain the capacity to see our modern-day emperors without clothes: they are not fooled by clichés, or the glitter of wealth, or power. Somehow they avoid being blunted by the process of so-called education. (For education, Kafka once remarked, means "probably but two things: First, the rebuttal of the children's impetuous assault on truth, and second, gentle, insidious, gradual initiation of the humiliated children into the lie." ["Wie ja allerdings wahrscheinlich alle Erziehung nur zweierlei ist, einmal Abwehr des ungestümen Angriffs der Kinder auf die Wahrheit und dann sanfte, unmerkliche, allmähliche Einführung der gedemütigten Kinder in die Lüge"; 1946.])

And, like many children, creative writers still feel the magic of words. To quote Simone de Beauvoir (1963): "Words vibrate in my mouth and through them I communicate with mankind. They relieve the arbitrary moment of its tears and transform the night and even death. It may well be my deepest wish that people will repeat a few words which I have linked." And, like many children, these artists appear to have a seemingly inexhaustible vitality, zest, and curiosity.

But being or remaining childlike is not enough. To become and stay creative, artists must possess an elusive commodity called "talent," and, even more important, they must be able to reconcile several structural contradictions that seem built into the creative process.

Thus, they must be able to pursue and mold their personal vision in the face of inevitable criticism, misunderstanding, or nonrecognition—and this the more so, the more novel and daring their vision. They must have a capacity for defiant loneliness, as it were, a basic, stubborn self-confidence which sustains them *coûte que coûte*. And yet they must reach out to others and must communicate their vision in ways which eventually will so grip or seduce these others that they come to share and appropriate it.

To achieve this reconciliation, artists must, as a rule, become totally absorbed in their private project, yet also must keep a foot in the public world; they must attune themselves to their unconscious processes to an unusual extent, yet must also check them against reality (or, better, against what others hold to be reality). In brief, they must use their creativity for the purpose of being with, as well as without, others, thus heeding Goethe, who said: "Man can find no better retreat from the world than art, and man can find no stronger link with the world than art."

Liberation from the Bad Mother and Family

To further explore this difficult venture of reconciliation, let me once more return to the toddler and his transitional objects. This toddler, we saw, liberated himself from his mother by packaging her desirable attributes into his blanket or teddy bear, while he got rid of undesirable ones. He creatively transformed his mother, as it were, as he split her up into several components, some good and retainable, others bad and disposable—as he made her movable and brought her under the spell of his imagination.

But such creative transformation of mother, we must now remind ourselves, has its limits—limits to be found in the child *and* in his mother. They are in the child insofar as his potential for creative liberation, while impressive, remains also precariously circumscribed. For whatever he does, he still needs his real mother (and will need her for a long time to come). He needs her protective shelter, her material and emotional nurture, her cognitive guidance; and, perhaps most important, he needs her to consider *him* important: he needs her to love him, not because he deserves it but because he is there, a little child.

This, then, brings into view those limits on his liberative efforts which are set by his mother—as when this mother fails to provide shelter, or fails to give proper nurture or guidance, or fails to bestow on him a deep sense of importance. When this happens, the child's plight worsens. Not only must he liberate himself from his (to use another term of Winnicott) "not-good-enough mother," but also, as much as he can, he must make up for her failings. He must become his own emotional repairman. He must find a creative solution not only to the dependence-independence dilemma, but also to his emotional deprivation, or harmful overstimulation, or mystification by his mother, or whatever the case might be.

Yet the mother, I must now add, while central to the child, is not all that counts. She is only part of the family which surrounds, sustains, and nurtures him. And while, in my *Conflict and Reconciliation*, published some five years ago (1969), I still focused almost exclusively on the mother-child relationship, I have by now become more "family conscious"; I have realized, for example, that the mother is often not the most mothering one in the family, or that she is often not the parent who offers the "strongest reality" (Stierlin, 1959), and that, therefore, many a child's efforts at liberation and repair are often directed chiefly to a parent or family member(s) other than his mother. Consequently, when we try to grasp the dynamics of such liberation, we must consider how the whole family stakes out an interpersonal arena of oppression and exploitation.

In the following, I want to take up two early transactional scenarios which may fatefully shape an artist's efforts at liberation and repair, and bear on his self-destruction. Elsewhere (1972b, 1973, 1974, and, with Ravenscroft, 1972) I have described these scenarios in detail. Here I must limit myself to a few orienting remarks.

Binding and Boundness

In one scenario, binding—or, if you wish, centripetal—
forces predominate. Here parents interact with their children
in ways that seem designed to keep the latter locked in the
family ghetto. The binding can operate on three major levels.
First, it can operate through the exploitation and manipulation of the child's dependency needs, as when he is infantilized
and offered undue regressive gratification. He is here doted on,
is kept in his sickbed when he should move out, is held back
from peers, and is spared age-adequate competitive challenges.[1]

Second, binding can operate on a more cognitive level,
where the parent, rather than guiding the child safely through
the everyday symbolic jungle, mystifies him about what he
feels, needs, and wants. This parent exposes a child to fuzzy
and contradictory messages, invalidates what the child perceives, attributes to him traits of weakness or badness,
misdefines him (the child) to himself, and fails to share with
him a "common focus of attention." L. Wynne (1963) and M.
Singer (1965), R. Laing (1965), G. Bateson (1969) with his
associates (1956, 1963), and P. Watzlawick et al. (1967),
among many others, have explored and articulated the
intricate dynamics of cognitive binding and boundness.

And finally, binding can operate on a third level where an
intense and archaic loyalty prevails. Unconsciously, the child
here views any separation from his parents, in thought or
action, as a murderous crime directed at them, for which only
the harshest punishment will do. Therefore he suffers an
enormous unconscious breakaway guilt that gives rise to acts
of either massive self-destruction or heroic atonement. In a
recent paper, reporting on my research with adolescents and
their families at the National Institute of Mental Health

1. In this context, see also Stierlin (1972a) and Stierlin, Levi, and Savard (1973).

(1973), I described how two deeply loyalty-bound youngsters engineered dramatic suicides in their attempts to cope with unbearable breakaway guilt.

Expelling and Waywardness

In the other transactional scenario—to be found at the other end of the scale—centrifugal and expelling forces predominate. Here parents neglect and reject their children, and the separation between the generations is aggravated. Rather than hanging onto their children for dear life and fostering a pathological loyalty, as happens within the binding scenario, such parents consider their children nuisances and human surplus to be gotten rid of.

The term *wayward* well describes what this implies for the children. For *wayward* derives from *awayward,* which means "turned away," and suggests expulsion as well as escape. The turned-away person is, according to the dictionary, self-willed, wanton, and prone to follow his or her own caprices. Along with that, he obeys no clear principle or law and often does the opposite of what is desired or expected.

Clearly, such waywardness, when extreme, precludes the kind of life most of us know and cherish. Nonetheless, many expelled, wayward persons exist and try to survive. For example, the Ik, a mountain tribe living in East Africa on the borders of Uganda, Kenya, and the Sudan, are described by the anthropologist Colin Turnbull (1972) as a people for whom extreme rejection and waywardness, as here defined, became a way of life. The Ik were originally nomadic hunters but were forcibly resettled. In this process they were uprooted, their social organization was shattered, and their traditional skills were made useless. *Homo* here soon became *homini lupus.* Even though the Ik shared a compound, each Ik was utterly alone in the world. Husband and wife went separately to search for food, never shared what they found, and—most important from my present perspective—drove their unloved

children out of their homes at the age of three. Turnbull
adduces example after example of this people's lack of loyalty
and concern, their egocentricity, and their imperviousness to
the needs of others, and he goes on to compare the Ik to the
inhabitants of modern ghettos, who also turn ruthlessness and
lack of concern and loyalty into assets for survival within the
metropolitan jungle.

Let us, then, examine how these two contrasting transactional scenarios may generate differing vicissitudes of liberation and creativity for certain artists. (Yet let us, in so doing,
also keep in mind that we may here easily go astray, as a great
artist's cosmos of experience is often so rich and complex that
we can find therein almost anything we want to find,
including the widest-ranging contradiction and paradox—
both seeming and real.)

The Writer's Liberation from Boundness

Some time ago (1972b) I wrote about Hölderlin, whom
many Germans consider their country's greatest poet. Hölderlin, I tried to show, was psychologically bound up with his
mother (the internalized, as well as actual mother), as he
sought her regenerative warmth yet at the same time courted
her deadly embrace. Finally, in trying to unbind himself, he
became mad and destroyed himself as artist. But even though
his liberation failed, he could analyze his plight. In one of his
letters he wrote: "from youth on I have reacted more
sensitively than other people to what could destroy me, and
this sensitivity seems to have to do with the fact that I,
considering the experiences I had to endure, became not
organized solidly and indestructively enough. So much I see.
But will that fact of seeing it help me? To this extent, I
believe: *Because I am more easily destroyed than other persons, I must
try all the harder to obtain an advantage from those things which have a
destructive influence on me.*" I know of no passage in literature
which so clearly states the promise, as well as perils, of a

liberation through creativity. But rather than expand on Hölderlin, let me turn to another bound-up writer, who seems even closer to us moderns—Franz Kafka.

Kafka, like Hölderlin, was no stranger to psychotic disintegration. Like Hölderlin, he possessed enormous gifts for self-analysis, for self-observation, and for precise, articulate description. And, like Hölderlin, he employed these gifts "to obtain an advantage from those things which" had a destructive influence on him—that is, those things that caused him to become and remain bound up. In using these gifts, Kafka managed to reconcile the seemingly irreconcilable in often stunning ways. One of the most private and autobiographical of writers, he yet captured the feelings that appeared most universal for his time—alienation and existential despair. While he seemed to lift his nightmares straight out of his unconscious, he yet chiseled them into masterful stories; and while he spoke like a religious prophet, he yet vibrated with subtle humor (so much so that Thomas Mann called him a "religious humorist"). But, rather than enumerate Kafka's creative reconciliations, let me take up some vicissitudes of liberation which he, a bound-up artist, exemplifies.

Binding, I said earlier, can operate on three major levels—a dependency level, a cognitive level, and an archaic loyalty level. What we know about Kafka from his many autobiographical stories, diary entries, and letters indicates that he was deeply bound up on *all* of these levels. He was bound up on the dependency level, as he received seemingly unending regressive gratification not only from his doting mother but also from his three sisters, particularly from Ottla, his favorite. Secondly, his father, an authoritarian bully, embodied not only the terror of castration but also willful arbitrariness. Kafka's famous letter to him, one of the most extraordinary psychological documents in literature, provides many examples of how this father—endowed with an "enigmatic innocence and inviolability"—mystified his son about what he (the son) felt, needed, and wanted, and thereby bound him to his (the father's) frame of reference. And thirdly, Kafka was deeply and pathologically loyalty-bound. Any attempt at self-assertion would therefore trigger a massive breakaway guilt that stymied him everlastingly in despair, self-flagellation, and self-blame. No wonder. Kafka could never marry, as marriage, while promising him the "most honorable independence," also posed the most deadly threat.

Kafka's writings convey this inextricable multilevel boundness. It pervades the nightmarish landscape of *The Trial* and *The Castle*; it pervades his letters and diaries; it pervades his conversations with friends. Also, it pervades his professional existence as a lawyer and employee in the Workmen's Compensation Office in Prague—for him a hated bureaucratic monster. (Because he saw bureaucracies as unshakable, he had no hope that social revolutions could succeed. Regarding the Russian Revolution, he mused, therefore: "As a flood spreads wider and wider, the water becomes shallower and dirtier. The revolution evaporates, and leaves behind only the slime of a new bureaucracy. The chains of tormented mankind are made out of red tape"—Janouch, 1971, p. 120.)

However, in the final analysis, it was not bureaucracies that chained Kafka, it was he himself. "I live in a cage," he tells the young poet Janouch, ". . . not only in the office, but everywhere . . . I carry the bars within me all the time" (Janouch, 1971, p. 20). And these psychological bars were made up of his lack of self-confidence, his sense of weakness, his fear of venturing into a cold, forbidding world strewn with innumerable traps and demands; but most of all, they were made up of his enormous sense of guilt over any possible liberative action or wish.

And yet Kafka struggled to liberate himself up to the last moment, making language, this "eternal mistress," the main ally, and his pen—"not an instrument but an organ of the writer"—the main weapon in this struggle. Kafka's whole state of being differed depending on whether he, at any given time, was able or unable to write. When he was unable to write, he was in deepest depression; he was, as he tells Felice Bauer, "at once flat on the floor, fit for the dustbin" (Kafka, 1973). It was then, observes Brod (1966), his long-term friend and biographer, "as if one looked into an abyss. But when he was writing, he seemed to burn from an innermost fire, even while under pain. Each time it was a miracle" (p. 109).

However, even the creative process with its miraculous energizing powers mired Kafka more deeply in his boundness, as he, like Hölderlin, tried harder and harder "to obtain an advantage" from those things which had a destructive influence on him, yet, also like Hölderlin, succeeded only in courting more destruction.

Two interweaving forces stand out here. First, Kafka's deep breakaway guilt annulled in the end all liberative gains from his writings. Thus, rather than making his writings into wings for a flight into freedom, he turned them into more fetters. No wonder, then, that he referred to these writings as mere "scribbling" *(Kritzeln)*, that he asked Max Brod to destroy all his manuscripts, that he became uncomfortable and embarrassed whenever people appreciated his works or alluded to his literary success. Therefore, I believe Kafka was right when he concluded that as "attempts at independence, attempts at escape," his writings met only "with the very smallest of success." Yet, even though they represented his only worthwhile attempts in this direction, he considered it his "duty or, rather, the essence of his life to watch over them, to let no danger approach them" (Kafka, 1953, p. 117).

To understand why his liberative efforts failed, we must also turn to the second major force which caused his downfall—the tuberculosis that finally killed him. To Kafka, the snorts and wheezes of the tubercular patient evoked the image of a beast that "bores its snout into the earth with one mighty push and tears out a great lump; while it is doing that I hear nothing;

that is the pause; but then it draws in the air for the new push. This indrawal of its breath which must be an earth-shaking noise, not only because of the beast's strength, but also because of its haste, its furious lust for work as well; this noise I then hear as a faint whistling. . . . Day and night it goes on, burrowing with the same freshness and vigor, always thinking of its objects. . . . Compared with this what are all petty dangers in brooding over which I have spent all my life?" (Kafka, 1948, p. 209). Kafka, clearly, tries to obtain an advantage even from his murderous illness by letting it generate a striking vision and by subjecting it to a penetrating psychological analysis; but in the end the "beast" wins out over all of Kafka's efforts to analyze, tame, and contain it. For, as the beast burrows deeper into his lungs, it saps Kafka's vitality and destroys his wish to struggle on, to seek independence, to marry. Finally, the only liberation he can envision is one of deep, regressive self-abdication—a liberation that amounts to a drift into nothingness and death.

When his tuberculosis was diagnosed on September 4, 1917, he wrote to his publisher, Kurt Wolff: "My illness, allured for years by headaches and insomnia, suddenly broke out. It is almost a relief" (Kafka, 1958, p. 159). This happened to be the moment when Kafka, after a deep inner struggle, was finally about to marry Felice Bauer. The sickness, noted his psycho-analytic biographer, John S. White (1967), now spared him this fateful act. It allowed him to quit his position at the Workmen's Compensation Office, which he hated so much. In addition, it allowed him to live with his sister Ottla, who managed a little rural boardinghouse in Zürau near Saatz. Hence the feeling of inner liberation, of quasi euphoria, that overcame him when he finally met his illness head on! Thus, the illness came at a time in his life when he was preparing to undertake what he held to be the most decisive step toward maturity—marriage; but rather than taking this step, he let himself, under the disguise of outer necessity, drift into passivity and ever deeper dependent boundness. He derived now from his tuberculosis, so he told Felice, "the kind of immense support a child gets from clinging to its mother's skirts" (Kafka, 1973, p. 545). And there was Ottla, a stand-in for his mother, ready to provide all the regressive gratification he could wish. "Ottla," he writes, "carried me so to speak on her wings, through a difficult world . . . the room is . . . excellent . . . all I am supposed to eat is here in big quantity and good quality (only the lips refused it in a spasm but this always happens in the first days of change) and the *freedom*, most of all, the *freedom*" (Kafka, 1958, p. 161). But clearly, this freedom was no longer the one he could hope to achieve through the creative process.

The Writer's Liberation from Waywardness

Where the second transactional scenario prevails, we must qualify the meaning of liberation. For the wayward expellee needs not so much freedom from, but a re-creation of and sharing in, human bonds—bonds that could nurture him, foster his loyalty and concern, and make him feel important. Therefore, the creative process—if it has a chance to operate at all—must aim here not so much at liberation from oppressive shackles, but at overdue repair work.

This task, however, is formidable. For we have good reason to believe that a rich maternal nurturing—a nurturing that has flowed at least somehow, sometime—is at the root of all later creativity. Therefore, too massive a deprivation and expulsion at an early age most likely kills the creative fire outright.

Still, where the expulsion has not been that massive, the creative flames may still burn. And it is here where even a wayward expellee, if he is creative, may "obtain an advantage from those things which have a destructive influence" on him—in other words, may obtain an advantage from his very expulsion and waywardness. Let us, then, look more closely at how he may do this.

Only recently I received an object lesson of how this might be possible. It happened while I was reading to my girls, ages 7 and 4, the stories of Pippi Longstocking, which a Swedish writer by the name of Astrid Lindgren (1969) created; for Pippi Longstocking is a wayward child whom her father, a vagabond sea captain, deserted. (She also seems to have lost her mother early.) This wayward Pippi turns her forced premature autonomy into an asset for survival, as she embarks on an unprincipled, willful, and unconventional life that unendingly fascinates masses of more conventional—that is, more restricted and bound-up—children. To their delight, Pippi goes to bed whenever she wants to, indulges in bad table manners, wears dirty clothes with holes in them, and does many other things which "nice" children just do not do. She also defies standards of conventional prettiness—she is red-haired, freckled, and rather skinny—and acts like a young protagonist of women's lib who thumbs her nose at a sexist, male-dominated society. Of course, it helps her that she can lift up a horse with one arm and hence can knock off boys by the dozen.

We have much reason to believe that Astrid Lindgren, in writing down Pippi's exploits, tried to master a difficult childhood fate, which probably was not one of bound-upness but one of early rejection and neglect—a fate which, I may add, seems rather common in Sweden. (For example, there we find lots of "key children," who are sent off to nursery school at the earliest possible moment, with a house or apartment key hanging around their necks, so as to allow their mothers a speedy return to their jobs. H. Hendin [1965], an American psychoanalyst, perceptively traced how such early neglect and rejection affects the personalities and relationships of Swedes.)

But children's stories à la Pippi Longstocking are one thing, and mature creative writings are perhaps another. Can writers of other than children's stories, we must ask, also obtain an advantage from the fact of their one-time deprivation and neglect? I believe this to be the case, and find that some of the dynamics of narcissism, as described by H. Kohut (1966), are illuminating here.

Certain so-called narcissistic individuals share some traits of wayward ones: they, too, were neglected and deprived as children, and they also seem impervious to the needs of others and, in following their own caprices, defy common values and principles. Interestingly—and my own observations agree with those of Kohut—not a few of them are unusually creative. Their creativity becomes at least partly understandable when we reason that the creative person must, first, be relatively free from conventions (i.e., free from ordinary regulatory expectations and principles), and that he, second, may have to seek his salvation through a precocious psychic synthesis and autonomy. In creating his own world or vision, he then "pushes"—frequently to the breaking point—his self-willedness and self-sufficiency.

Typically, many of these narcissistic individuals have on the surface an excessive sense of self-importance; closer inspection, however, reveals the very opposite—namely, a lack of a sense of self-worth and a desperate defense against the threat of being found insignificant. It is this threat which turns such persons' endeavors into one relentless quest for the confirmation of their importance (an importance that they inwardly doubt), a quest which fuels, as well as colors, their creative processes.

Such self-willed and self-seeking or, if you wish, narcissistic artists are in some respects better off than bound ones like Kafka. By exploiting their narcissism and maintaining their freedom from commitments, they also safeguard their creativity. Bertolt Brecht, while not necessarily belonging to this group, seemed nonetheless to speak for it when he said: "In me

you have one on whom you cannot rely" ("In mir habt ihr
einen, auf den könnt ihr nicht bauen"). And they appear
neither weighed down by massive breakaway guilt nor
aggrieved over hurting or exploiting others, as others have
meaning to them only in terms of fulfilling their needs and/or
serving their quest for importance. Totally absorbed in their
creative ventures, they recruit these others either as un-
swerving admirers or as living, externalized fantasies who are
discarded once they have fulfilled their purpose and who are
not recognized by the narcissists as persons with rights, needs,
and interests of their own. Therefore, it need not surprise us
that many of these creative artists operate in human disaster
areas that are strewn with the wreckage of ruined lives and
hopes.

Interweaving of Danger and Salvation

But just as a bound artist appears to be in constant danger
of losing his creative edge in despair, so does one who is bound
too little. Whereas the former may confront the deeper sources
of his creativity too closely and vulnerably, the latter may lose
touch with them altogether. Sooner or later his narcissistic
aloofness may cause him to dry out, as he protects himself too
successfully from human interactions, and hence from the
experience of dependency, conflict, and guilt—the stuff of
which life's drama is made.

The German poet Stefan George, whose narcissism impressed many of his contemporaries, reflects such a drying-out
process. Born in 1868, he published six books between 1890
and 1900. Thereafter his productivity began to wane and
ceased altogether around 1920. He died in 1933. What he said
about Nietzsche seems to describe George himself during his
last decades:

> Thou killed yourself what thou held nearest,
> To, newly longing, tremble after it

And cry out loud in loneliness and pain.[2]
[My translation]

In the light of the above, it is not surprising that liberation through creative work seems to fail as often as it succeeds, be the artist bound-up or narcissistically alienated. A. Alvarez (1973), who had his own bout with suicide, reminds us of the enormous casualty rate among artists in this century. He states:

> Of the great premodernists, Rimbaud abandoned poetry at the age of twenty, Van Gogh killed himself, Strindberg went mad. Since then the toll has mounted steadily. . . . Virginia Woolf drowned herself, a victim of her own excessive sensitivity. Hart Crane devoted prodigious energy to aestheticizing his chaotic life—a desperate compound of homosexuality and alcoholism—and finally, thinking himself a failure, jumped overboard from a steamer in the Caribbean. Dylan Thomas and Brendan Behan drank themselves to death. Antonin Artaud spent years in lunatic asylums. Delmore Schwartz was found dead in a run-down Manhattan hotel. Joe Orton was murdered by his boyfriend, also a writer, who then committed suicide. Cesare Pavese and Paul Celan, Randall Jarrell and Sylvia Plath, Mayakovsky, Esenin and Tsvetayeva killed themselves. Among the painters, the suicides include Modigliani, Arshile Gorki, Mark Gertler, Jackson Pollock and Mark Rothko. Spanning the generations was Hemingway, who . . . in the end . . . followed the example of his father and shot himself. [pp. 228–29]

This is a long list, and it could easily be expanded. And yet,

2. "Du hast das nächste in dir selbst getötet
   Um neu begehrend dann ihm nachzuzittern
   Und aufzuschrein im schmerz der einsamkeit"
   (1907, p. 232).

while it shows that that which may save the artist—namely, the creative process—may also destroy him, the reverse is equally true: in the words of Hölderlin, "along with the danger, salvation is also forthcoming" ("mit der Gefahr wächst das Rettende auch").

To make this final point, let me share with you what Simone de Beauvoir writes at the end of her three-volume autobiography (1963). She reflects here on her increasing age (and her childlessness), which weighs her down, saps her vitality, and ensconces her in a lonely, melancholy prison; yet then she goes on:

> The moment a writer writes, he gains a chance to escape petrification. With each new book, I set a new beginning. I doubt, I lose courage, the work of past years is wiped out, my notes appear so unusable that I think it impossible to finish my project—up to that elusive moment . . . when it becomes impossible *not* to finish it. Each page, each phrase requires then a new imagination, a total resolve. Creative work is adventure, is youth, is liberation. [p. 616]

REFERENCES

Alvarez, A. *The Savage God.* New York: Bantam Books, 1973.

Bateson, G. "Double Bind, 1969." Presented at Symposium on the Double Bind, annual meeting of the American Psychological Association, Washington, D.C., Sept. 2, 1969.

Bateson, G.; Jackson, D.; Haley, J.; and Weakland, J. "Toward a Theory of Schizophrenia." *Behavioral Science* 1 (1956) :251–64.

———. "A Note on the Double Bind." *Family Process* 2 (1963): 154–61.

de Beauvoir, S. *Der Lauf der Dinge.* Translated by P. Baudisch. Reinbeck: Rowohlt, 1970. [*La Force des Choses.* Paris: Gallimard, 1963.]

Brod, M. *Der Prager Kreis.* Stuttgart: W. Kohlhammer, 1966.

Hegel, G. *The Phenomenology of the Mind,* 2 vols. Translated by J. B. Baillie. London: Swann Sonnenschein, 1810.

Hendin, H. *Suicide and Scandinavia.* New York: Doubleday-Anchor, 1965.

Janouch, G. *Conversations with Kafka. Notes and Reminiscences.* New York: New Directions, 1971.

Kafka, F. *Beschreibung eines Kampfes/Novellen, Skizzen, Aphorismen aus des Nachlass.* New York: Schocken, 1946.

———. *Diaries.* Edited by M. Brod. Vol. 1, 1910–1913. Vol. 2, 1914–1923. New York: Schocken, 1948.

———. *Letter to His Father.* New York: Schocken, 1953.

———. *Letters.* New York: Schocken, 1958.

———. *Letters to Felice.* New York: Schocken, 1973.

Kekulé, A. *Theoretical Organic Chemistry. Papers Presented to The Kekulé Symposium* (1865). London: Butterworths Scientific Publications, 1959.

Kohut, H. "Forms and Transformations of Narcissism." *Journal of the American Psychoanalytic Association* 14 (1966): 243–72.

Laing, R. D. "Mystification, Confusion, and Conflict." In I. Boszormenyi-Nagy and J. L. Framo, eds., *Intensive Family Therapy.* New York: Harper & Row, 1965.

Lincke, H. "Wirklichkeit und Illusion." Unpublished manuscript, 1973.

Lindgren, A. *Pippi Longstocking.* New York: Viking, 1969.

Singer, M. T., and Wynne, L. C. "Thought Disorder and Family Relations of Schizophrenics. III. Methodology Using Projective Techniques. IV. Results and Implications." *Archives of General Psychiatry* 12 (1965): 187–212.

Stierlin, H. "The Adaptation to the 'Stronger' Person's Reality." *Psychiatry* 22 (1959): 143–52.

———. *Conflict and Reconciliation.* New York: Doubleday-Anchor (paperback); Science House (hard cover), 1969.

———. "Family Dynamics and Separation Patterns of Potential Schizophrenics." In D. Rubinstein and Y. O. Alanen, eds., *Proceedings of the IVth International Symposium on Psychotherapy of Schizophrenia.* Amsterdam: Excerpta Medica, 1972(a).

———. "Lyrical Creativity and Schizophrenic Psychosis as

Reflected in Friedrich Hölderlin's Fate." In E. E. George, ed., *Friedrich Hölderlin, An Early Modern.* Ann Arbor: University of Michigan Press, 1972(b).

Stierlin, H. "A Family Perspective on Adolescent Runaways." *Archives of General Psychiatry* 29 (1973): 56–62.

———. "Hitler: A Family Perspective." Monograph in preparation, 1974.

Stierlin, H., and Ravenscroft, K., Jr. "Varieties of Adolescent Separation Conflicts." *British Journal of Medical Psychology* 45 (1973): 299–313.

Stierlin, H.; Levi, L. D.; and Savard, R. J. "Centrifugal Versus Centripetal Separation in Adolescence: Two Patterns and Some of Their Implications," in S. Feinstein and P. Giovacchini, eds., *Annals of American Society for Adolescent Psychiatry.* Vol. 2, *Developmental and Clinical Studies.* New York: Basic Books, 1973.

Turnbull, C. *The Mountain People.* New York: Simon & Schuster, 1972.

Watzlawick, P.; Beavin, J. H.; and Jackson, D. D. *Pragmatics of Human Communication.* New York: Norton, 1967.

White, J. S. "Psyche and Tuberculosis: The Libido Organization of Franz Kafka." *Psychoanalytic Study of Society* 4 (1967): 185–251.

Winnicott, D. W. "Transitional Objects and Transitional Phenomena. A Study of the First Not-Me Possession." *International Journal of Psycho-Analysis* 34 (1953): 89–97.

———. "The Location of Cultural Experience." *International Journal of Psycho-Analysis* 48 (1967): 368–72.

Wynne, L. C., and Singer, M. T. "Thought Disorder and Family Relations of Schizophrenics. I. A Research Strategy. II. A Classification of Forms of Thinking." *Archives of General Psychiatry* 9 (1963): 191–206.

4

August Strindberg's Need-Fear Dilemma, as Seen in His Relationship with Harriet Bosse*

DONALD L. BURNHAM AND SVEN ARNE BERGMANN

In the course of several years of research on schizophrenia, one of us (DLB) focused on several particular aspects of this complex illness or syndrome: for one, the patient's relationships; for another, his patterns of thought and communication. Relationships are of key significance at various points in the schizophrenic process. First, disordered relationships contribute to the development of a personality vulnerable to schizophrenia; second, disordered relationships are a major symptom; and third, relationships are an important agent in treatment.

The schizophrenia-vulnerable person suffers an extreme form of a perhaps universal human conflict—the need-fear dilemma—which dominates his relationships with other persons. He is, at one and the same time, enmeshed in an inordinate need for, susceptibility to, and fear of, the influence of others. As a result, it is enormously difficult for him to establish a stable and comfortable closeness-distance balance in his relationships. If too close—he disorganizes; and if too distant—he disorganizes. He tries to attenuate his dilemma through various combinations of clinging to and avoiding other persons, and distorting his percepts of them.

* A version of this paper in Swedish appeared in *Meddelanden från Strindbergssällskapet*, no. 50, May 1972.

73

The need-fear dilemma is linked to key personality deficiencies that are the result of faulty development and that result in a weak and easily disorganized ego, the central system of control and organization. The normal ego integrates personality subsystems into a harmonious whole. It provides relative, not absolute, autonomy from two sets of demands: those of inner forces, such as drives and affects, and those of the external environment. An ego lacking this degree of autonomy is excessively vulnerable to influence and upset by both sets of demands, and the person has difficulty in regulating himself. For want of reliable internal structure, he both needs and fears regulation from without.

These formulations were derived primarily from clinical studies of schizophrenia (Burnham et al.). Another remarkably illuminating source is to be found in the writings of August Strindberg, the Swedish playwright, for whom recognition and appreciation lagged in the United States until recent years.

The need-fear dilemma is a salient theme in Strindberg's writings and life. He was a tortured man who dwelt on the border of schizophrenia and during several life crises was in danger of slipping over that border. Diagnostic judgment must necessarily be tentative when one knows a person only from writings by and about him. However, it appears probable that Strindberg's personality was seriously vulnerable to schizophrenia, though it seems doubtful that he ever suffered fragmented disorganization. Certainly he never underwent anything resembling mental deterioration. He did manifest many paranoid traits which, in combination with his genius for verbal formulations, probably enabled him to reshape experiences and to organize reality in a manner that protected him from fragmented disorganization. Periodic withdrawal into relative solitude and communion with nature doubtless also helped him to avoid gross disorganization. Even during his most disturbed periods he retained an awesome mastery of language and the ability to make his meanings crystal clear, despite the dubiousness of some of the premises from which he reasoned.

Perhaps it is fair to say that Strindberg several times approached the abyss of schizophrenia, close enough to look searchingly into the turmoil therein but without ever plunging over the precipice. Out of these experiences he was able to report invaluable insights into the dynamics of the schizophrenia-vulnerable personality. With his exquisite sensitivity and verbal genius he could report in a way seldom, if ever, possible for persons who have actually gone over the brink into chaos.

These insights pervade the more than sixty volumes of his writings. However, in this paper we shall focus principally upon two sets of documents, his letters to Harriet Bosse, his third wife, and portions of the so-called *Occult Diary*, which he kept during their brief marriage and for several years thereafter. During that time Strindberg managed a partial resolution of his need-fear dilemma. After separation he and Harriet continued to correspond and to see each other quite regularly; to a degree this was a satisfactory closeness-distance balance for both of them. In many respects writing afforded him a much more satisfactory mode of communication than face-to-face talk. Entries in his diary were perhaps even easier, since if he chose, no one need ever see it.[1] Communication at a distance was analogous to his fondness for his telescope, which during his Blue Tower[2] years provided him with a *sense* of close contact with others without the danger of actual closeness. Doubtless the letters, and more particularly the diary, comprised multiple levels and nuances of meaning for both Strindberg and Harriet. In addition to their interpersonal communicative significance, they afforded him a vehicle for inner dialogue and for giving shape and expression to inchoate feelings.

1. His indecision and repeated changes of mind about its eventual publication are well known.

2. The Blue Tower was his nickname for the apartment building in Stockholm where he lived the last four years of his life. It now houses the Strindberg Museum.

Strindberg's need-fear dilemma was manifest in his relationships not only with people but also with ideologies and belief systems. His need impelled him to seek sustenance, completeness, unity, purity, and harmony in closeness to other persons and to ideologies. Yet closeness inevitably aroused his fear that others would weaken, contaminate, and destroy his self. These fears in turn generated defensive hatred. This relentless sequence of need and fear drove him through countless cycles of attraction and repulsion, of idealization and disillusionment, of belief and cynicism, of mythopoesis and mythoclasm.

These patterns can be seen with special clarity in his three torturously unsuccessful marriages. The popular notion of Strindberg as a misogynist is a gross oversimplification. He was as much a woman-worshiper as a woman-hater. He looked to each of his wives for far more than relief from loneliness; he envisioned their bringing him redemption, salvation, healing, and purification. He yearned to be cleansed of his hatred and distrust and thereby reconciled to life and humanity and freed to create goodness and beauty in his writings.

Strindberg's imagination irresistibly constructed utopian visions of an ideal woman rescuer leading him to a better, higher life. Of course, the real outer world repeatedly failed to live up to the ideal of his inner world. Idealization was inexorably followed by disillusionment. Withal, he never fully relinquished his quest for the ideal rescuing woman. Even in his final year of life, he seriously considered marrying Fanny Falkner, a teen-aged actress.[3]

In envisioning the ideal woman, Strindberg gave free rein to romantic and poetic flights of fancy, which sometimes extended to idiosyncratic and autistic perceptions and restructurings of reality. He also had recourse to a private lovers'

---

3. One is reminded of the shipwrecked mariner in the title role of *The Dutchman*, who, despite the failure of six marriages, is advised by his mother, "Search and do not give up" (the quest for redemption by a woman), and who then embarks on a seventh marriage (see "Le Hollandais," p. 47).

language. He fervently sought a woman of constant purity who would evoke only pure love. Thus he hoped to escape the waves of fear, disappointment, and hatred that incessantly threatened to overtake and engulf him. The snag was that the idealization process overlooked and attempted to bypass very real imperfections and inconsistencies in the other person. More important, by idealization he tried to deny and circumvent the deep ambivalence and inconstancy of his feelings toward women. Relationships established on this basis were not likely to endure.

His letters to Harriet Bosse and his *Occult Diary* provide vivid descriptions of the idealization-disillusionment sequence which marked the failure of Strindberg's effort to overcome his need-fear dilemma by marrying her. This occurred despite his desperate struggles to integrate his feelings and to resolve his conflict as to whether outer reality would confirm or contaminate his ideal images.

Strindberg and Harriet were married in 1901 and divorced in 1904, but between those dates they actually lived together only briefly and intermittently. They were married on May 6. His diary entry for May 7 was the single word, "Harmony." On May 8, however, he wrote of longing to run away and of beginning suspicions and dissensions. A series of quarrels, separations, and reunions paralleled the oscillations of his feelings. When they were together, he devalued her; when apart, he idealized her. Here is his description: "There is a woman whom I cannot bear to be near, but who is dear to me at a distance. We write letters, always appreciative and friendly; but after we have longed for one another for a time and feel we must meet, we instantly begin to quarrel, grow coarse and disharmonious, part in anger. We love one another on a higher plane, but are not able to be in the same room and we dream of meeting again, disembodied, on a verdant island where only we two may be and, at most, our child" (*Diary*, p. 9).

From the outset, Strindberg's relationship with Harriet seems to have been more with his image of her than with her actual self. He first saw her while seeking an actress to play the leading role of the Lady in his strongly autobiographical play *To Damascus Part I.* At the time, three possible candidates for the role were appearing in *A Midsummer Night's Dream.* Harriet, an ingenue of twenty-one, was acting Puck. Despite her youth and inexperience, Strindberg chose her for the role of the Lady.[4]

Strindberg chose Harriet not only for this role in his soon-to-be-produced play, but even more important, for the role of ideal woman in his fantasy of being rescued from his emotional torments—all this without much actual contact with her. His vision of her contained elements that he himself considered strange, supernatural, and mystical and that an objective observer might consider autistic expressions of Strindberg's intense emotions.

At the first dress-rehearsal of *To Damascus* in November 1900 they met for perhaps the third time, and Strindberg confided to his *Occult Diary*: "First dress rehearsal of *Damascus.* The inexplicable scene with (Bosse). It happened like this! After the 1st act I went on to the stage and thanked (Bosse). Made some comments about the final scene where the kiss has to be given with veil down. As we stood there on the stage, surrounded by a lot of people, and I was talking seriously to her about the kissing scene (Bosse's) little face changed, grew

4. Quite possibly the bisexual implications of her playing Puck may have influenced his choice. In the *Occult Diary* (p. 16) he recorded a dream: "I was lying in a bed, B came to me in her Puck's costume from the play. She was married to me. She said of me: 'Behold, the man who brewed me,' and gave me her foot to kiss. She had no breasts, absolutely none!"

Another possible determinant of his initial attraction to Harriet might be that in 1900 she also had acted Anna in Gustav Wied's *The First Violin.* Anna was the name of Strindberg's favorite sister, to whom he was deeply attached; his *Occult Diary* (p. 16) notes that his nephew had seen Harriet in *To Damascus* and had said that she resembled Anna Strindberg Philp.

larger and became supernaturally beautiful, seemed to come closer to mine while her eyes enveloped me with their luminous blackness. Whereupon, without excusing herself, she ran away and I stood amazed, feeling that a miracle had happened and that I had been given an intoxicating kiss.

"After this (B) haunted me for three days so that I could feel her presence in my room" (pp. 15–16).

At the end of the two weeks' run of *To Damascus* early in December, Strindberg sent roses to Harriet and noted in his diary, "with thorns, of course—they say there are no others!" In addition to commenting on life in general he seems, perhaps, to be hinting at the mixed quality of his emerging feelings toward Harriet.

A week later he wrote in his diary, "Fancied I was having telepathic relations with (B)" (p. 17). Then in his diary entry for January 13, 1901, he wrote, "(B) . . . haunted me on the 12th. This haunting grew more intense on the 13th, and at night she persecuted me. . . . When she appeared telepathically during the night I 'possessed' her. Incubus" (p. 18).

By mid-February he wrote, "Night before: uneasy. Woke at 2 o'clock. *(Possessed her when she sought me.)* My telepathic relationship with (B) has intensified alarmingly. In my thoughts I live solely with her. *(Pray God to resolve this matter.)* It threatens to bring about a catastrophe" [5] *(Diary*, p. 22).

During the time that the relationship was reaching this pitch of intensity in his dreams and fantasies, their contacts in shared reality were rather few and far less sensational. She came for an occasional meal at his apartment, but most of their communication was via letters. On the surface these letters mostly concerned Strindberg's reading and writing, though often when he spoke of characters in his plays, he was referring symbolically to himself and Harriet. On a photo of

5. The italicized words in parentheses were written in Greek characters in the original diary, presumably a partial effort at disguise.

himself he inscribed, "To the 'Lady' from the 'Unknown One' " (principal characters of *To Damascus*; *Diary*, p. 25).

He asked her to play the leading role in several plays he wrote during this time, including *Easter* and *The Bridal Crown*. Partly to help Harriet prepare for the role of Eleanora in *Easter*, Strindberg sent her several books. He especially wanted her to read a Kipling story, "In the Land of Dreams" (in some editions, "The Brushwood Boy"). Kipling tells of a boy and girl who meet only once in childhood, but who later as adults realize that during the intervening years they have been close companions in shared dream adventures. On this basis, after only two or three actual meetings, they decide to marry, a sequence not dissimilar to what happened between Harriet and Strindberg.[6]

During one of Harriet's actual visits he asked for and received an eagle feather from her hat, with which to make a quill pen to use in writing his plays. Very probably this had powerful symbolic overtones, including the wish that she act as his muse and give him permission and inspiration to wield his pen.[7]

Meanwhile, what Strindberg took to be telepathic contacts intensified further. He was convinced that he could sense her presence in his room by odors, which he associated with sexual temptation and concern as to how his body smelled. He found himself using a photo of her to stimulate erotic fantasies, but

6. On Feb. 24, 1899, Strindberg had written to his literary colleague Geijerstam, "I was frightened when I read *The Brushwood Boy* because the author believes in it and so tricks the reader into believing" (Lamm, p. 409).

7. The eagle had deep and multiple significance for Strindberg. Fellow members of the Runa Society of his student days had given him the nickname of "the eagle," and he sometimes signed letters with this sobriquet. A stuffed eagle was a companion during his Blue Tower years. He identified with the eagle's proud independence and flight high above the earth, but was less accepting of the eagle's predatory way of life. On the occasion of his engagement to marry Harriet, he wrote her a poem which began, "To Harriet/(written with the eagle pen)/Fear not the eagle, pure white dove!/never—oh beloved!—will he rend you" (*Letters . . . to Harriet Bosse*, p. 27).

after kissing the picture he would be flooded with guilt and shame for his "evil thoughts." He was relieved to mail her photo to a friend in Germany with the hope that it might help her obtain acting engagements there. On another occasion he tried to fight temptation by throwing her picture into a closet.

He spoke in his diary of urges to flee to Paris or Berlin, or to a monastery in Italy, but was unable to muster the resolve to actually do it, just as years before he had started on an abortive trip to Paris in an effort to escape emotional entanglement with a married woman, Siri von Essen, who subsequently became his first wife. The idea of monastic retreat had intrigued Strindberg off and on for several years. In a letter to his painter friend Richard Bergh, concurrent with his excitement and alarm over his telepathic contacts with Harriet, he wrote that he was planning to relieve others of the "irritating" presence of his "bulky, untidy person" by departure for a monastery (Lamm, pp. 360–61).

On the other hand, he invited Harriet to urge him not to leave. According to his diary entry of March 2, 1901 (p. 31), he had asked her, "Ought I to let 'the Unknown One' end up in a monastery?" and she had answered, "No, he has more to accomplish in life." Though ostensibly asking her how to end *Damascus III*, a draft of which he had sent her a few days before, he was also appealing, "Please ask me to stay and to marry you."

Unable to trust his own feelings to resolve his indecision, Strindberg looked to the outside for guidance. For the answer to the question of whether he and Harriet were in love he looked for omens and signs, even in such trivial, everyday events as the brightness of the sky on certain days, the pattern of light on his bed covers, or the stopping of his watch at a certain hour. In anticipation of one of her actual visits to his apartment he thought, "now I have her in a trap," but when she arrived looking childlike and gentle, he heard warning rapping noises in all the walls (*Diary*, p. 31). When he began to

consider remarriage, he assumed that a cut on his ring finger
was another possible warning (*Diary*, p. 22).

His belief that his personal destiny was in the hands of
outside powers is vivid in this diary entry (pp. 22–23):

> What I am now going through is horrible and marvel-
> lous—I feel as if I were expecting a death-sentence.
> Sometimes I think that *(she loves me)*, sometimes not.
> God's will be done! If I only knew what it was. Up to now
> there have been as many premonitory signs for as against.
> On her last visit I felt as if an angel were in the room and
> I decided in favour of the good; hoping to achieve
> reconciliation with woman through woman. For three
> days now I have had her in my room and experienced an
> elevating, ennobling influence, which surely no demon
> could possess.
>
> If the Supreme Powers are jesting with me, I am
> prepared to bear that too!

Among the most important of omens to him were smells,
whether actual or imagined. The smell of celery and unclean
sexuality were linked, as were incense and purity. The smell of
incense convinced him of Harriet's telepathic presence. But at
times the smell seemed unpredictably to change to something
nauseous and terrifying. He prayed for her guardian angel to
make her good and to make him good through her. Then,
seized by doubt, he would wonder whether his angelic image
of her was a delusion. He told himself, "Demons can dress up
like angels" (*Diary*, p. 24).

Finally he managed to declare his feelings to her, though
exactly when and how are not entirely clear. According to
Harriet's subsequent recollection, "He told me how severely
and harshly life had treated him, how much he longed for a
ray of light, a woman who could reconcile him with mankind
and with woman. Then he laid his hands on my shoulders and
looked deeply and ardently at me and asked, 'Will you have a

little child by me Fröken Bosse?' I curtsied and answered quite
hypnotized, 'Yes, thank you,' and then we were engaged"
(*Diary*, p. 34).

During their two months' engagement period, Strindberg,
for the most part, saw Harriet as an angelic rescuer, as in this
passage from a letter:

> "To me you are 'Swanwhite', and when last night I laid
> my great terrestrial-globe of a forehead beneath your
> little celestial one, then I knew that the universe had
> fallen into a state of harmony, and I noticed how I, an
> earth-spirit, was winning heavenwards through you, a
> spirit of the air!
>
> "This had to be written, for I could not say it. Hide it,
> for it is true, truer even than reality, knowledge, or
> experience!" [*Diary*, p. 35]

Now and then, when other feelings intruded, Strindberg tried
to attribute them to the workings of outside powers, witness
this example:

> "Forgive me, friend, for disturbing your enjoyment yester-
> day, but there are certain Forces over which I have no
> command.
>
> "As long as I stay peacefully at home, I have calmness,
> the moment I go out and mingle with people, the Inferno
> begins. That is why I long for a home of my own!"
> [*Letters*, p. 31]

His reluctance to share her company with others, coupled
with his fear of contact with outsiders, foreboded trouble, and
Harriet voiced her fear of becoming a prisoner. He countered,
however, that it was more likely that he, the eagle, would be
caged by her. It did not take long after marriage for this
problem to become acute. He resented her going out, and
when her sister, Dagmar Möller, introduced her to other men
he referred to Dagmar as a "procuress" (*Diary*, p. 37). When

Harriet wanted to go to a masked ball, Strindberg bought trunks and threatened to leave.

He proposed a European trip together but at the very last moment called it off, and groaned, "We are not going, the Powers will not allow it" (*Diary*, p. 39). According to Harriet, he then gave her a Baedeker so she could take an imaginary trip without the troubles of an actual journey. He counted it preferable to see people at a distance than to be in their actual midst (*Letters*, p. 42).

Soon thereafter Harriet took off alone for Denmark, without at first telling him her destination. When he learned her whereabouts, he wrote a mixed acknowledgment and denial of a sense of loss: "After having wept in my retreat, which I have not been outside for three days, I received your letter. . . . My dearest! Can you not feel at a distance—distance is something that does not exist for us—that I am living only in you, that I love you? You are with me all the day long, and the incense of your being sweeps to me here through space . . . I no longer see you in the flesh . . . I see only your soul, its beauty and goodness—which you were beginning to forswear" (*Letters*, pp. 44–45).[8]

A few days later Strindberg joined her for a month in Denmark. Then, after a brief, upsetting visit to Berlin, they returned to Stockholm, where it was confirmed that Harriet was pregnant. This news precipitated intense quarrels. Probably both of them were highly ambivalent about having a child. Strindberg spoke of her "sorrowing over your lost youth which I have 'laid waste' " (*Letters*, p. 53). When she said that the child would be named Bosse, not Strindberg, he reacted with pain and fury, and saw her transformed from an angelic rescuer into a hateful poisoner. Her pregnancy stirred several

8. Harriet sometimes contributed to his belief in telepathic contacts, as when she wrote, "My thoughts follow you, as always. Oh that I could slip into your new home with them" (*Diary*, p. 53).

other complicated emotional undercurrents in him. These included: guilt about their sexual activity, which the arrival of a child would announce to the world; envy of his wife's procreative capacity; and whisperings of rivalrous wishes to be her only love, if not her only child.

He now found himself flooded with precisely those feelings from which he had sought rescue: guilt, envy, and hate. In his diary he wrote, "I feel that my spirit is bound down to the lower spheres of activity where my wife now operates" (p. 47). And in a letter he wrote: "the yellow room[9] became malodorous. It was your selfish hatred that gave out the stench—it was not I" (*Letters*, p. 54). The result was another sequence of separation and reunion.

Almost a year later Strindberg was able to interpret some of his feelings in a letter written to Harriet while she was away in the country with their daughter: "And in my aloneness I have you with me; but with others around you, you disappear from view, and the contact ceases. What was our disagreement about? Yes—about keeping our own individuality when we were in danger of melting into one. . . . It made me feel horror-stricken at times, having surrendered myself so unconditionally to you. I wanted to flee, but I could not. All this is quite natural, as natural as that love has a seeding and a blossoming time. One yearns for the seed, but feels the loss of the flower when the seed has come" (*Letters*, pp. 84–85).

Subsequent events after their separation and divorce, and especially after Harriet became engaged to Gunnar Wingård (1908), revealed even more clearly the large autistic component in Strindberg's relationship with her. He was convinced that she contacted him telepathically almost nightly and made passionate sexual advances to him. In his *Occult Diary* he spoke of sensing her presence by a smell or a taste: pleasant (roses) if she were friendly, unpleasant (formalin) if she were angry.

9. The "yellow room" was his term for Harriet's bedroom.

When his heart palpitated, he believed that she must be excited or anxious. He attributed abdominal tension and pain to movements of her uterus within his belly. (Example: "A sort of dragging sensation began in the small of my back and proceeded downward through my pelvis on the opposite side. I assumed from this that Harriet was about to start her period. This was confirmed later on by the fact that she only sought me shyly and without delight. We wrestled amiably until the morning, when I was victorious"—*Diary*, p. 119.)

To the degree that he was convinced of the reality of his telepathic contacts, Strindberg could overlook whether actual contacts confirmed or refuted his beliefs. His private reality was more malleable than shared reality. He could deny the painful reality of humiliation, loss, and separation. After learning of Harriet's engagement to another man, he wrote in his diary: "She becomes engaged to W., but at night she flies to me. We live as if we were newly married" (p. 114). In another apparent effort to deny his loss, he proposed that they have another child.

Harriet's efforts to break off actual communication appear to have been sufficiently ambivalent and ambiguous to leave some room for Strindberg's belief in continued telepathic contacts. However, her fiancé did write a threatening letter telling Strindberg to stop persecuting her. By way of response Strindberg wrote in his diary: "For the whole of today, since the stroke of 5 this morning, we have lived as one; the same heart-beats, the same sufferings, the same fears! Now she is at the theatre, acting before the public, but she is with me! Talking to me. Never can we part" (p. 138).

To buttress his denial, he sometimes resorted to splitting his image of Harriet. For instance, when told by a friend that banns for Harriet's remarriage had been published, he was stunned and asked himself, "Is she literally two persons? And do I possess one? The better one?" (*Diary*, p. 129). By splitting, he endeavored not only to deny painful hurt but also to explain and justify his deep ambivalence toward women, which, of course, long antedated his relationship with Harriet. Another splitting device was to assume that Harriet awake was drastically different from Harriet asleep, as in this diary note: "At times she seems to seek me in her sleep. When I wake and respond, she wakes up and withdraws. This makes it appear as if when unconscious (sleeping) she wants to possess me, but when conscious does not!" (p. 124). Of course, it was actually *he* who was different when asleep.

Some of Strindberg's ideas about the capacity of the soul to become "exteriorized" and to travel telepathically through space were derived from Swedenborg, and also from occultist writers whom he had read in Paris during his Inferno period.[10] Such beliefs nicely fitted his efforts to account for the apparent changeability of other persons and of his feelings toward them.

A good example of his disclaiming responsibility for his ambivalence is seen in this diary entry: "Woke again at about 6 in a violently erethistic state. Wanted to take her in my arms then and there, but was instantly disarmed. This suggests that during my sleep, she is within my body, but when I wake she withdraws, for otherwise this sudden retreat on my part is inexplicable. Such a thing usually takes time, but this happened in an instant. It used to be the same in our conjugal life when she sought me and offered herself; but as soon as I came to her I was deprived of my arms by her 'Athanor,' which seemed to possess an individuality of its own" (p. 133). Here Strindberg split his ambivalence between Harriet and her "Athanor," his term for her uterus.[11]

10. In addition, for several years he studied psychological writings, particularly those concerned with suggestion and hypnosis, techniques by which one person could exert powerful influence over another even at a distance. Somnambulism and dreams and the possibility of awakening to other levels of consciousness and reality were related topics of immense fascination for him.

11. He was familiar with the word *athanor*, an alchemist's furnace, from his earlier preoccupation with alchemy; it probably also is linked to his rivalry with his wives as to whether he or they were the more truly creative. In writing about the womb in *A*

The issue of the extent to which he could exert conscious control over not only body parts and processes but also thoughts and fantasies was almost an obsession with Strindberg. Often he believed that he, and humanity at large, must act according to a script written by Higher Powers. At other times he ventured to consider himself the scriptwriter. Rather than allowing Harriet to write *fini* to their relationship, he asked a producer to stage *Swanwhite*, his earlier betrothal gift to Harriet, with her and her new fiancé in the principal roles (*Diary*, p. 112).

In another twist of the denial process, Strindberg asserted that Harriet was going to marry, not another man, but an offshoot of his (Strindberg's) soul *in* the other man: "Fortunately I have never seen him, but yesterday I saw a photograph [of him]! He resembled me; but his self was dead—and he had become so much like me that he seemed an offshoot of my soul—from playing my plays and from associating with you! He was I—I in the large portrait of myself—I in all my youthfulness. I did not begrudge you that youthful appearance of his in preference to my older appearance. But he himself was dead!" (*Letters*, p. 174).

The depth of Strindberg's conviction of the reality of his telepathic contacts was variable. Sporadically, he tried to rationalize them in spiritualistic, pseudoscientific, or supernatural terms, but he seems never to have believed completely in Swedenborgian or occultist systems of thought. Sometimes he referred to an "illusion" of Harriet's presence, but at other times he seemed more convinced of the reality of the experience. He even wondered

> if there will not emerge from our supernatural marriage small beings of a spiritual nature . . .

Blue Book, Strindberg said, "It resembles the alchemist's Athanor, in which were distilled the Philosopher's Stone, gold, the Elixir of Life, and the homunculus" (*Diary*, p. 130 n). Other writers, too, have linked the womb, the alchemist's vessel, and the poet's imagination—for example, "Mallarmé is the alchemist; he does not find the stone, but he stumbles, in his search for it, on such fascinating compounds that we are very willing, in Donne's phrase, to glorify his pregnant pot" (Kermode, p. 115).

Whatever happens I shall learn of it through my own sensations for the soul of your body is in mine. [quoted in *Diary*, pp. 126–27]

Another day, while reading of Swedenborg's belief in a double existence in different realities, Strindberg began to wonder, "whether H——t is conscious of our life together, or whether the personality I embrace is a 'double' about whom she knows nothing, a phantom" (*Diary*, p. 148).

In *A Blue Book*, dedicated to Swedenborg, Strindberg had already made a penetrating analysis of how a relationship can be complicated when one person constructs unverified, autistic percepts of the other:

When a man begins to love a woman he throws himself into a trance, and becomes a poet and artist. Out of her plastic, unindividualised material he fashions an ideal form into which he puts all that is best in himself. Thus he creates an homunculus which she adopts as her double, and with that she lets him do as he likes.

But this astral image may be also the doll which she the huntress sets up as a decoy, while she with a loaded gun lies behind the bush and watches for her prey. The love of a man for his homunculus often survives every illusion; he may have conceived a deadly hatred against herself, while his love for her double continues. But this masquerade gives rise to the deepest dissonances and troubles. He becomes squint-eyed by contemplating two images which do not coincide. He wishes to embrace his cloud, but takes hold of a body; he wishes to hear *his* poem, but it is someone else's; he wants to see his work of art, but it is only a model. He is happy during his trance, although the world cannot understand him. When he awakes from his somnambulism, his hatred to the woman increases in proportion as she fails to correspond to his image of her. And if he murders her double, then love is done with, and only boundless hate remains. [*Zones of the Spirit*, pp. 216–17]

Strindberg was uncertain about where to allocate the blame for the failure of the real person to match his ideal image. Sometimes he blamed the other person, as when he wrote to Harriet: "Why did you not wish to be what I created you to be in my imagery? I could not have pulled you down, as you said! That I don't believe!" (*Letters*, p. 169). At other times he blamed third parties, who he thought exerted contaminating influence either by their actual presence or by evil thoughts. Occasionally, in a more reconciled mood, he blamed life itself. After rereading some of their correspondence, he wrote to Harriet, "I find in these letters the very finest in us, our souls in holiday dress, as life in the flesh seldom is . . . in your letters you live and reveal yourself as 'the great woman' I suspected you to be. That the every-day type does not fulfill these characteristics is the fault of life itself, which is so grim and which provides such unlovely situations" (*Letters*, p. 171).

Increasingly he returned to the idea that life may be a dream through which we move like sleepwalkers and that only in death will we awaken to true reality. He had said earlier, during the second major separation from Harriet, "We do not belong here and we are too good for this miserable existence. . . . Life, for me, was as unmanageable as a woman" (*Diary*, pp. 47–48). Contributing to the unmanageability was not only the ideal-real discrepancy but also the fact that direct proximity to the real person inevitably triggered the return of affects and impulses that he had tried to repress and eliminate by creating the fantasied ideal, which remained adorable only from a safe distance.

Strindberg yearned to be purged of deep fear, distrust, and hatred: "You have taught me to speak with purity, to speak beautiful words. You have taught me to think loftily and with high purpose. You have taught me to forgive an enemy. You have taught me to have reverence for the fates of others and not only my own" (*Letters*, p. 37). When the actual woman failed to purify him, he could write: "We are absolutely forced to do evil and to torment our fellow men. It is all sham and delusion, lies, faithlessness, falsehood and self-deception. 'My dear friend' is my worst enemy. Instead of 'My beloved' one should write 'My hated' " (*Diary*, pp. 76–77).

Sometimes Strindberg's fear of the dirtiness of hatred appears to have assumed very literal forms. Harriet stated that during arguments he "would go over to a wash basin in his room and wash his hands hastily, nervously, again and again" (*Letters*, p. 80). Sexual urges were another problem which he seemed unable to resolve by either distance or closeness, because his own inner conflict about sex remained unresolved. In writing of his first telepathic "intercourse" with Harriet, he said, "The whole thing seemed to me quite ghastly and I *(begged God to deliver me)* from *(this passion)*" (*Diary*, pp. 18–19). His reading about Indian religions led him along a line of philosophizing which echoed his personal conflicts about sex:

> The primary Divine Power (Maham-Atma, Tad, Aum, Brama) allowed itself to be seduced by Maya, or the Impulse of Procreation.
> Thus the Divine Primary Element sinned against itself. (Love is sin, therefore the pangs of love are the greatest of all hells.)
> The world has come into existence through Sin—if in fact it exists at all—for it is really only a dream picture . . . a phantom and the ascetic's allotted task is to destroy it. But this task conflicts with the love impulse, and the sum total of it all is a ceaseless wavering between sensual orgies and the anguish of repentance. [*Diary*, p. 55]

Doubtless Strindberg's abortive urge to enter a monastery partly represented a wish to escape sexual temptation. He voiced fears both of besmirching the innocent woman and of

being contaminated by her. Here is an example of the latter:
"I don't know why I feel animosity when you show friendliness
in a particular way. . . . Do not touch my fate with wanton
hands! How often didn't I warn you? But you—in your
arrogance—had to do it—like the rest!" (*Letters*, p. 97). One of
Harriet's letters seems further to confirm the relentlessness of
Strindberg's sexual guilt: "I must not be together with you any
more for the reason that—should we come together again—
you will see it as something unbeautiful. Oh, it is that, of
which I am afraid!" (*Letters*, p. 71).

One attempted effort to relieve his conflict was to attribute
it to her, as in this diary entry: "Impossible to know where you
are with women. Whatever you do is wrong. One day they call
you a *(satyr)*, the next day a *(Joseph)*. You can never tell what
they want, if they are *(sensual)* or *(chaste)*" (p. 48). Although it
is quite probable that Harriet actually had sexual conflicts, it
would appear that, here, Strindberg was indulging in defensive projection.

His wish to escape this conflict was also evident in his desire
for a purely spiritual relationship, something akin to the
sexless love of angels as extolled by Swedenborg. In part, but
only in part, he preferred telepathic to actual sexual intercourse. Witness this outcry: "It was my soul that loved this
woman, and the brutalities of marriage disgusted me. For that
matter, I have never really been able to understand what the
not very elegant act of procreation has to do with love for a
beautiful female soul. The organ of love is the same as one of
the excretory organs" [12] (*Diary*, p. 47). Even before their
marriage Strindberg had expressed a premonitory latent wish
for a distant type of relationship, when he wrote to Harriet: "If
it is the will of Providence—well then we shall part as friends
for life; and you will remain my immortal faraway Love, while

---

12. A sentiment echoed in Yeats's lines, "But love has pitched his mansion in/The
place of excrement" (*Collected Poems*, p. 254).

I shall be your servant Ariel, watching over you from afar! I shall warm you with my love and my benevolent thoughts. . . . I shall protect you with my prayers!" (*Letters*, p. 37).

Another aspect of Strindberg's sexual conflicts was his dread that his private life might become public knowledge. He accused Harriet of having given away the secrets of the "Yellow Room" (*Letters*, p. 52). Strindberg's wish that third parties not be privy to his intimacy with Harriet had other important ramifications, including intense jealousy. He wanted her for himself alone. Once, in a restaurant, when an officer at a nearby table glanced a few times at Harriet, Strindberg became furious and insisted that they leave immediately (*Letters*, p. 39). When a photographer snapped a picture of Harriet at the seashore, Strindberg struck the man on the head with his walking stick (*Letters*, pp. 45–46). This jealousy extended to a dread that, through her, other persons would enter into intimate contact with him; witness these diary entries:

> I feel defiled through her. Unknown men defile me by the glances with which they defile her . . . if she is free and has an affair with another man, she delivers over my soul and transmits my love to that man, and thus forces me to live in a forbidden relationship with a man's soul or body or both. [pp. 46–47]

Subsequently, when Harriet became engaged to Gunnar Wingård, Strindberg's fear of homosexual contact became still more intense, as is attested by this excerpt from his letter of April 11, 1908, to Harriet:

> Of one thing I am certain; I shall not survive your wedding night, not out of envy, but because of the power I have of imagining what will take place.
> So be it! On that night I shall celebrate my marriage with death! God will allow me that after all my suffering!

> For I must go before my true self, my immortal soul is defiled. It is no good my saying to myself: Why should he touch my woman? She is not mine in the ordinary sense, and he has the right. But she is my creation, all the same, and there is in her something of me for him to touch . . . it is me he caresses, that is why I must depart!
>
> Why will you not let me go? What do you want with my old person? Take my soul if you must, but let me go! This will end badly! [quoted in *Diary*, p. 113]

The idea that he had deposited parts of his self, if not of his soul, in Harriet was linked to another of the fears which closeness to others aroused in Strindberg. This was the dread of losing his self, his independent identity, to the other person—a protean dread. He feared the influence of others, in whatever form it might be exerted; he was constantly on guard lest others exploit him and steal his physical and mental resources. Moreover, he feared the loss of his self-possession and self-control. His dread arose not so much from the predatory, domineering propensities of other persons as from the intensity of his own dependent yearnings. He felt that surrender to these yearnings would render him a helpless child or slave. Accordingly, it was difficult for Strindberg to accept help either gracefully or gratefully, and he tended to turn against benefactors and to transform them into enemies. The same can be said of his tendency constantly to seek advice but to distrust all advisors (Lamm, p. 298).

Assir's statement in *Isle of the Dead* could well have been uttered by Strindberg about himself: "Oh, I exist all right; I react to others. And if I stopped doing that, the others would engulf me with their egos, their opinions, their fancies. They'd kill me with their will; I should cease to exist. The whole struggle of my life has been to preserve my ego!" [13] (Vowles, p.

13. This is perhaps an appropriate point at which to say something about the relationship between Strindberg's life and his works, and the importance of his

377). And directly to Harriet he wrote: "You Black Swanwhite! You took with you all my good thoughts, took them
away. Now take with you everything, everything, the child
too. And go!" (quoted in *Diary*, p. 118).

In *Damascus III* the Stranger tells the Lady, "You have
sucked the marrow out of me, eaten me hollow, killed
everything within me—my very self, my personality!" (p. 312).

Strindberg's conflict about closeness also extended to the
fantasy of fusion with others—craved as a means to unity and
completeness but equally dreaded as a threat to separate
individuality. This is perhaps the deepest level of the need-fear
dilemma. As noted above, he gave it eloquent expression in a
letter to Harriet: "What was our disagreement about? Yes—
about keeping our own individuality when we were in danger
of melting into one" (*Letters*, p. 84). In *Damascus III* the
Stranger says, "Ours is not an ordinary love. We are like two
drops of water that are in fear of coming too close . . . lest
they should cease to be two and turn into one" (p. 313).

Though somewhat eased in his final years, Strindberg's
dilemma never became fully resolved. Basically, he remained
trapped in the pattern he once described to Harriet: "My
discordant emotions tear me apart; my loneliness drives me to
seek people out, but each time—even after a most genial
contact—I withdraw injured and hurt and find myself still
more depressed" (*Letters*, p. 129). The inexorability of this
dilemma tempted him repeatedly to withdraw from actual

---

imagination in both. We do not subscribe to the notion that Strindberg's writings can
be treated largely as thinly disguised autobiography. Though certainly he reworked
life events in his writings, the creative product is far more complicated than a direct
mirroring or reporting of these events.

His extraordinary imaginative abilities were of great significance in both his work
and his life. Although for his work his imagination was a tremendous asset, it was not
always so in his life, where it often was a source of misunderstanding and discord in his
actual relationships with other persons. We believe that he struggled mightily to try to
maintain control over his imagination, and over his ability to test reality and to
distinguish between the creatures of his imagination and creatures of other origins.

contacts in shared reality and to try to construct with his imagination a more ideal world. In *The Great Highway*, one of his last plays, he wrote:

> Beauty does not exist in life,
> cannot materialise down here.
> The ideal is never found in practice.

And in these lines from the same play, he imparted his dream of perhaps finding his ideal in death:

> For the last time I strip
> and go to rest, to sleep—
> And when I wake—my mother will be there,
> my wife, my children, and my friends.

[p. 679]

REFERENCES

Burnham, Donald L.; Gladstone, Arthur I.; and Gibson, Robert W. *Schizophrenia and the Need-Fear Dilemma*. New York: International Universities Press, 1969.

Kermode, Frank. *Romantic Images*. New York: Vintage, 1957.

Lamm, Martin. *August Strindberg*. Translated and edited by Harry G. Carlson. New York: Benjamin Blom, 1971.

Strindberg, August. *From an Occult Diary: Marriage with Harriet Bosse*. Edited by Torsten Eklund, translated by Mary Sandbach. New York: Hill and Wang, 1965.

———. *The Great Highway*. In *Twelve Plays of Strindberg*, translated by Elizabeth Sprigge. London: Constable & Co., 1963.

———. "Le Hollandais." Translated by C. G. Bjurström. *La revue théâtrale*, vol. 9, no. 30 (1955).

Letters of Strindberg to Harriet Bosse. Edited and translated by Arvid Paulson. New York: Thomas Nelson & Sons, 1959.

Strindberg, August. *Queen Christina*. Translated and introduced by Walter Johnson. Seattle: University of Washington Press, 1955.

———. *Swanwhite*. In *Twelve Plays of Strindberg*, translated by Elizabeth Sprigge. London: Constable & Co., 1963.

————. *To Damascus III*. In *Eight Expressionist Plays by Strindberg*, translated by Arvid Paulson. New York: Bantam Books, 1965.

————. *Zones of the Spirit: A Book of Thoughts*. Translated by Claud Field. London: George Allen and Co., 1913.

Strindberg, Frida. *Marriage with Genius*. Translated by Frederic Whyte from *Lieb, Leid und Zeit*. London: Jonathan Cape, 1937.

Vowles, Richard B. "Strindberg's 'Isle of the Dead.' " *Modern Drama* 5 (1962–63): 366–78.

Yeats, W. B. *Collected Poems*. New York: Macmillan, 1952.

Psychiatry, Philosophy, and the Development of Thought

5

The Mystical Experience of the Self and Its Philosophical Significance*

> "Soul is a being that can be beheld by God
> and by which, again, God can be beheld."
> —Hadewijch, Letter 18

Louis Dupré

Much of what is written in the philosophy of religion deals with abstract generalities and makes exceedingly tedious reading. It is as if philosophers had not yet learned to apply to religion what they do as a matter of course in the area of science: to acquaint themselves thoroughly with the subject. Since this subject includes full rational articulation as much as prereflective experience, it requires a detailed study of *particular* theologies. Religious categories are not transhistorical concepts: they originate in specific religious cultures and develop with those cultures. What we need, far more than the current analysis of presumably universal concepts, is a philosophical equivalent of Bremond's *Histoire littéraire du sentiment religieux*. This is particularly true for the entire area of mystical experience and its systematic expression. Here more than anywhere else the principle holds: there is no mysticism, there are only mystics and specific mystical theologies. This is not to deny the existence of a common element in the variety of

* Louis Dupré's essay, written for this volume, also appeared in *International Philosophical Quarterly*, December 1974. Reprinted by permission.

experience—indeed, one of philosophy's main tasks is precisely to discover this element—but in the actual texts in their historical setting.

The significance of such a study is not restricted to the sole area of philosophy of religion. It would affect other, more general philosophical notions that have developed on the basis of a too limited reflection. A primary instance is that of the notion of the *self*. Philosophy, particularly empiricist philosophy, has largely been satisfied with describing and cataloguing the content of the ordinary consciousness. But some suspected long ago that there might be more to the self than what the unperceptive eye so easily detects. In his distinction between "apperceptions" and "petites perceptions," Leibniz attempted to go beyond consciousness by introducing elements which, although not fully conscious themselves, nevertheless play a constitutive role in consciousness. His simple juxtaposition of both elements is inadequate to explain the *structure* of selfhood; yet it reveals an amazing awareness of the difficulty created by the interrupted consciousness (in states of sleep or sickness) for any theory which attempts to interpret the self as a string of phenomena united by means of a common memory. Memory itself, in spite of total discontinuity, is what most urgently needs to be explained. To bridge the gaps of consciousness the self clearly requires a subphenomenal dimension.

William Ernest Hocking was one of the few to heed this requirement. Interestingly enough, he was led to do so by reflecting on the religious concept of immortality.[1] He posits two "selves," one conscious of the world in which it lives (the excursive self), the other transcending the worldly flux and thereby enabling the other self to become conscious (the reflective self). The reflective self is not subject to the lapses of the excursive one: steadfastly it maintains itself through the

1. William Ernest Hocking, *The Meaning of Immortality in Human Experience* (New York: Harper, 1957), pp. 44–59.

blackouts of consciousness and connects the intermittent stretches of consciousness. The body may be an indispensable instrument in this constant process of identification, but it cannot provide its ultimate foundation, since the body itself needs to be recognized as identical from one stretch to another. The self, then, surpasses the sum total of psychic phenomena. Indeed, the phenomena themselves remain unintelligible unless we accept a subphenomenal source from which they spring and which gives them their coherence. The founding self depends considerably less upon its bodily environment than the phenomenal self. The former's activity continues uninterruptedly after a withdrawal from the physical world in sleep, in trance, in artistic creation, or even in daydreams. Particularly in the latter two states, we notice a strange interference of the unconscious with the conscious self. On such occasions, the self appears to be led beyond the boundaries of its ordinary world and to escape its ruling laws. It becomes expressive rather than reactive, revealing the workings of an inner power instead of those of its bodily world.

Such a view is, of course, not new in modern philosophy. It was anticipated in Kant's transcendental ego, Fichte's pure "I," Schelling's Absolute, and, more recently, in Husserl's transcendental reduction. Yet on the whole, philosophers have seldom attempted to give this deeper self a positive content and, in the case of Kant and his followers, have explicitly denied that such a content could be given. The subphenomenal self remained mostly a condition of the phenomenal self.

Indeed, the exploration of the self as it extends beyond consciousness has been done outside the realm of philosophy proper. Whatever little scientific knowledge of it we possess, we owe to the psychological investigations of conscious behavior that could not be explained in terms of consciousness alone. Unfortunately, the therapeutic success of depth psychology has become one of the main obstacles preventing a full theoretical exploration of the unconscious self. The unconscious part of the self is obviously more than a storage place for what the mind has forgotten or blocked out. Nor must it be regarded as merely the more "primitive" part of the self, in which the more instinctual conflicts take place. Primitive it may be, in the sense in which the "lower" is said to precede the "higher."

> What we call subconsciousness, far from being a sort of mental sub-basement, is at the center of selfhood, and the invidious term "subconsciousness" is an inept recognition of the fact that the primary springs of selfhood are not habitually at the focus of its outgoing interests.[2]

Nor can one unqualifiedly maintain that a self which is not conscious cannot be known and is therefore no legitimate object for discussion. Although the unconscious as such undoubtedly escapes the direct glance of perceptive awareness, it may well manifest itself indirectly, as the achievements of depth psychology have proven. Moreover, those who have reached for the most intensive experience of the self have at all times believed that they would attain in the end a self no longer circumscribed by the bounds of ordinary consciousness. The very purpose of the mystical journey is to surpass consciousness and to rest in the dark source of the conscious self.

If we may attach any credence to the revelations of the mystics—and the universal nature of their experience forces us at least to consider their claims seriously—an altogether different layer of selfhood hides beneath the familiar succession of outward-orientated phenomena. Behind the gates to this restricted area the laws ruling ordinary consciousness seem to be suspended. Space and time recede or are transformed from a priori forms of outward perception into vistas of an inner realm with unknown rhythms and successions. From archaic depths the imagination (if it has not taken leave

2. Ibid., p. 50.

altogether) conjures well-structured visions known to the dream consciousness only through fragments, and to the waking consciousness not at all. In privileged instances the intellectual intuition, so peremptorily exorcised by Kant's critique, reasserts its rights, and the mind literally *perceives* as directly as the senses ordinarily do. The intellectual visions described by John of the Cross and Ignatius of Loyola are truly *visions* in that they belong to the order of perception even though all sensory input and perhaps all images have been halted. Does all this not support William James's observation that the ordinary, rational consciousness is only one kind of consciousness, while all around it, separated from it by the flimsiest screens, there are potential forms of consciousness of a completely different nature? To James the psychologist a full knowledge of the self requires the contribution of the peak religious experience.[3]

The Religious Origin of the Concept of Soul

The exceptional character of the mystical experience tempts us to isolate it from all others. But if its vision is unique, its foundation is not. For the mystical experience merely brings to full awareness the common religious principle that the soul itself rests on a divine basis. To the religious mind the soul is always more than it is—it transcends itself—so that the way inward must eventually become the way upward or downward (depending on the schema one adopts). This transcendence becomes manifest in the mind's self-understanding when the ordinary consciousness starts loosening its grip. At this point, religious man claims, we enter the sanctuary where God and

3. Obviously, I do not accept Erich Neumann's interpretation of the mystical types as corresponding to the three stages of life ("Mystical Man," in *The Mystic Vision*, ed. J. Campbell [Princeton, N.J.: Princeton University Press, 1968]). Such a reductionist projection is the exact opposite of what I have in mind. Instead of subsuming the unknown under the known, I want to expand the known by *adding* the novel *in its own right.*

the soul touch. It is also the very core of the self, as Meister Eckhart so daringly expressed:

> There is something in the soul so closely akin to God that it is already one with Him and need never be united to Him. . . . If one were wholly this, he would be both uncreated and unlike any creature.[4]

To lose one's God, then, is to lose one's deepest self, to become "unfree" and to be reduced to a "substance," a part of the world. Only in its capacity to transcend itself does the soul's power to surpass the world altogether lie. The religious mind will find it symptomatic that even a creative theory of man, such as Marx's was, runs into difficulties with a concept of freedom that lacks true transcendence.

The concept of soul is originally a religious one. According to Tylor's theory, religion originates with the awareness of a ghost-soul that is able to wander away while the body remains stationary, and that eventually will leave the body altogether. Although Tylor's simplistically evolutionist and intellectualist interpretations of the primitive mind were later rejected, on one crucial issue he was undoubtedly right: the idea of soul itself emerges as a religious notion and remains so, long after it has ceased to be primitive. Plato's view that the soul longs to rejoin the divine forms to which it is related sinks its roots into primary beliefs that long preceded philosophical reflection. Most North American Indians believed that the soul was created separately by a god. Aake Hultkranz, the Swedish student of native American religions, does not hesitate to generalize:

> As a rule, the Indians of North America believe that man's spirit has its ultimate origin in the deity himself, either through creation or partial emanation. . . . A soul

4. *Meister Eckhart*, trans. Raymond Bernard Blakney (New York: Harper, 1957), p. 205.

that is commonly considered to derive from the gods is *ipso facto* not an ordinary profane creation. Whether it is conceived to be a gift of the deity or an emanation of his being, it belongs through its origin to the supernatural world. The supernatural origin of the human soul finds particularly clear expression in the idea of pre-existence.[5]

We find similar concepts among Australian natives. To the Murngin tribe, the soul is what lifts man above the profane existence and allows him to participate in the sacred values of an eternal civilization.[6] In the Greek mystery cult the soul is above all a subject of ecstasy, first in this life and eventually in the afterlife.[7] According to Rohde, the awareness of this ecstatic quality is what led to the belief in immortality.[8] The notion of a substantial soul itself may have been born out of the ecstatic experience and the concomitant belief in immortality.[9] In any event, it is certain that the archaic notion of the soul is mainly characterized by what Rudolf Otto calls "the element of feeling—stupor—which it liberates, and the character of 'mystery' and 'wholly otherness' which surrounds it." [10]

Even developed religious cultures have preserved this numinous quality. Thus, much in the Upanishadic movement may be regarded as an attempt to penetrate that point of the soul where Atman is Brahman. The absolute is what I am in my true self: *Tat tvam asi*. The Bhagavad Ghita describes the

5. *Conceptions of the Soul Among North American Indians* (Stockholm, 1954), pp. 412–24.

6. W. Lloyd Warner, *A Black Civilization* (New York: Harper, 1964), p. 436.

7. Wilhelm Bousset, "Die Himmelsreise der Seele," *Archiv. für Religionswissenschaft* 4 (1901): 253 ff.

8. Erwin Rohde, *Psyche*, trans. W. B. Hillis (New York: Harper Torchbooks, 1966), pp. 264, 291.

9. Th. K. T. Preuss, *Tod und Unsterblichkeit in Glauben der Naturvölker* (1930), p. 17; cited in Gerardus Van der Leeuw, *Religion in Essence and Manifestation* (New York: Harper Torchbooks, 1963), p. 311.

10. Rudolf Otto, *The Idea of the Holy*, trans. John Harvey (New York: Oxford University Press, 1958), p. 194.

Atman in terms of the sacred: "marvelous," [11] "indestructible," "immutable," "incomprehensible." [12]

Christian theology regards the soul as created and is therefore more reserved, at least in its orthodox expression. Yet by no means did it "desacralize" psychology. The concept of the soul as an image of God determines the development of Christian mysticism as much as the notion of the Atman determines the Vedantic vision. The divine "character" of the redeemed soul, clearly present in St. Paul, was developed into a Christian psychology by the Cappadocians in the East and by St. Augustine in the West. The religious origin of their theories makes us all too easily overlook their psychological significance. To Gregory of Nyssa and Augustine, the fundamental structure of the soul can be understood only from a transcendent perspective. Thus the first theologies of the soul were also the first attempts at depth psychology. Nor should we dismiss them as purely theoretical speculations. Whatever the quality of their interpretations may be, they were primarily attempts to articulate and to justify an *experience*.

The Deeper Self of the Mystics

In accordance with the principle stated at the beginning of this paper, I shall abstain from attributing more than a "characteristic" or typological significance to each particular mystical description of the self. Nor do I expect my elementary remarks in any way to disclose the phenomenological *essence* of the experiences. At this initial stage of what Whitehead called the "descriptive generalization," I feel unable to do more than

11. *The Bhagavad Ghita*, trans. Eliot Deutsch (New York: Holt, Rinehart & Winston, 1968), 2, 29, p. 49. R. C. Zaehner translates the term *ascaryam* (marvelous) as "*by a rare privilege* may someone behold it" (New York: Oxford University Press, 1969; p. 50), while Rudolf Otto reads "*as wholly other* does one gaze upon it" (*Idea of the Holy*, p. 195).

12. *Bhagavad Ghita*, 2, 17–18, p. 38. A similar idea is expressed in the *Visnu-smrti* 20, 53.

to point out some striking differences between the ordinary self and the mystical self.

In fact, the very existence of an essential difference presents the most salient point in mystical literature on the soul. Thus, Ruusbroec clearly distinguishes the mystical awareness from the ordinary one: in the former, reason is suspended and the mind is emptied of all objects.

> Here our reason must be put aside, like every distinct work; for our powers become simple in love, they are silent and bowed down in the presence of the Father. This revelation of the Father, in fact, *raises the soul above reason, to an imageless nakedness.* The soul there is simple, pure and spotless, empty of all things, and it is in this state of absolute emptiness that the Father shows his divine brightness. To this brightness neither reason nor sense nor remark nor distinction may serve; *all that must remain below;* for the measureless brightness blinds the eyes of the reason and compels them to yield to the incomprehensible light.[13]

A difference between two levels is universally suggested by metaphors of isolation, secrecy, height, and, of course, depth. St. Teresa speaks of the inner castle, Catherine of Siena of the interior home of the heart, Eckhart of the little castle, Tauler of the ground of the soul, the author of *The Cloud of Unknowing* of the closed house, Plotinus of the innermost sanctuary in which there are no images.[14] St. John of the Cross combines several metaphors in the second stanza of his famous poem:

> In darkness and secure
> By the secret ladder, disguised—oh happy chance—
> In darkness and in concealment
> My house being now at rest.[15]

13. *Een Spieghel der Eeuwigher Salicheit,* in *Werken* (Tielt, 1947), 3:212.
14. *Enneads* VI, 9, 11.
15. *Dark Night of the Soul,* in *The Complete Works of St. John of the Cross,* vol. 1, trans. E. Allison Peers (New York: Doubleday, 1959), p. 34.

Omnipresent are images of depth.[16] Almost equally common is the image of height. The soul must "ascend" beyond images and understanding. In Plotinus this metaphor dominates, and the term *beyond* is the most significant one in the *Mystical Theology* of Pseudo-Dionysius, his Christian interpreter.

What characterizes the new state of consciousness above all is its qualitative distinctness. Ordinary psychic activity ceases to function and the mind is "taken" into the ground of itself, to which it has no independent access. In the *Katha Upanishad* we read:

> Atman is not to be obtained by instruction,
> Nor by intellect, nor by much learning.
> He is to be obtained only by the one whom he chooses;
> To such a one Atman reveals his own essence.[17]

Even the most cautious interpreters speak of "passive" states and "infused" contemplation. In the so-called quietist school, passivity became the overriding characteristic of spiritual life.[18] In some texts of the Vedanta this mental passivity appears to exclude consciousness. Thus, in the *Brhad-Aranyaka Upanishad* we read:

> As a man, when in the embrace of a beloved wife, knows
> nothing within or without, so this person, when in the

16. William Johnston describes the mystical process, in *The Cloud of Unknowing*, as a descent to "the still point or the ground of the soul," in which "the mind goes silently down into its own center, revealing cavernous depths ordinarily latent and untouched by the flow of images and concepts that pass across the surface of the mind." *The Still Point. Reflections on Zen and Christian Mysticism* (New York: Harper & Row, 1971), p. 132.

17. R. E. Hume, *Thirteen Principal Upanishads* (New York: Oxford University Press, 1931), *Katha*, 2, 23, p. 350.

18. One of the propositions endorsed by Molinos and condemned by Pope Innocent XI reads: "Doing nothing the soul annihilates itself and returns to the source and origin, the essence of God, in which it remains transformed and deified. God remains in Himself because then there are no longer two things united but one sole thing. In this way God lives and reigns in us and the soul annihilates itself in the very source of its operations." Denzinger-Bannwart, *Enchiridion Symbolorum* #1225, trans. Elmer O'Brien in *Varieties of Mystic Experience* (New York: Rinehart, Holt, 1964), p. 304.

embrace of the intelligent soul, knows nothing within or without.[19]

But no description ever surpassed the one found in the Mandukya of the fourth state of being, beyond dreamless sleep, in which all awareness of world and multiplicity totally vanishes.[20] Those texts originated in a tradition that does not mince words when emphasizing the distinction between mystical and ordinary states of consciousness. Yet Christian writers, though more moderate in their expression, also strongly contrast the ways of discursive knowledge with the modes of contemplation. The entire Neoplatonic tradition, which directly or indirectly includes most of Western mysticism, is expressed in Dionysius' paradox:

> Into this Dark beyond all light, we pray to come and, unseeing and unknowing, to see and to know Him that is beyond seeing and beyond knowing precisely by not seeing, by not knowing.[21]

John Tauler equally stresses the discontinuity with ordinary thought.

> This inner ground of the soul is only known to very few people . . . it has nothing to do with thinking or reasoning.[22]

St. Augustine's distinction between the discursive *ratio* and the *intellectus* that is directly illumined by God's light,[23] was to be

19. *Brhad-Aranyaka* 4, 3, 21; Hume, p. 136.

20. *Mandukya* 5; Hume, p. 392.

21. *Mystical Theology, Migne,* P. G. III, 1000. Trans. Elmer O'Brien, in *Varieties of Mystic Experience,* p. 83.

22. *Sign Posts to Perfection. A Selection from the Sermons of Johann Tauler,* ed. and trans. Elizabeth Strakosch (St. Louis: Herder, 1958), pp. 95–96.

23. *In Joan. Evang.* 15, 4, 19. On this distinction, cf. Etienne Gilson, *The Christian Philosophy of St. Augustine,* trans. L. E. M. Lynch (New York: Vantage Books, 1967), p. 270.

adopted by numerous spiritual writers after him. Richard of
St. Victor describes the mystical ecstasy as a state of consciousness in which the soul is "cut off from itself." [24]

The Ligature of the Faculties

As reflection on the distinct states of consciousness increased, a theory of the activity of the "faculties" in the
mystical consciousness emerged. In *Dark Night of the Soul*, St.
John describes the transition from the ordinary to the spiritual
level:

> In this state of contemplation which the soul enters when
> it forsakes meditation for the state of the proficient, it is
> God who is now working in the soul; *He binds its interior
> faculties* and allows it not to cling to the understanding,
> nor to have delight in the will, nor to reason with the
> memory.[25]

St. Teresa frequently refers to the paralyzation of the ordinary
psychic functions, as in the following passage:

> When all the faculties of the soul are in union . . . they
> can do nothing whatever, because the understanding is as
> it were surprised. The will loves more than the under-
> standing knows; but the understanding does not know
> that the will loves, nor what it is doing, so as to be able in
> any way to speak of it. As to the memory, the soul, I
> think, has none then, nor any power of thinking, nor are
> the senses awake, but rather as lost.[26]

24. On the basis of the Vulgate translation of *Hebrews* 4:12, he distinguishes
between *anima* and *spiritus*. Cf. *Selected Writings on Contemplation*, ed. and trans. Clare
Kirchberger (London: Faber and Faber, 1957), p. 204.

25. *Dark Night of the Soul*, 1:9, 7. Peers trans., p. 67.

26. *Relations* IV.

The preceding texts must not be understood to mean that all
"faculties" ceased to function at once. We notice St. Teresa's
hesitation when she comes to memory. A nineteenth-century
spiritual writer states explicitly: "The soul's powers are not
always in the same degree of drowsiness. Sometimes the
memory remains free, with the imagination." [27] Most of the
time the "faculties" do not cease to function at all. They are
"bound," which means that they no longer function in the
ordinary way. The Spanish mystics insist that the will always
continues to function, even though free choice no longer
exists.

But, above all, mystical states remain states of awareness,
namely, cognitive states. Some mystics, especially in the
Dominican school, consider ecstasy primarily an intellectual
act, though not a discursive one. By several accounts the
imagination and the senses also may become endowed with
new powers. Thus the mystic in certain cases *sees* visions and
hears voices, either with the senses or the imagination, which
others do not perceive.[28] Are sensations that are not supported
by ordinary sensory stimuli simply "illusions," as the term
hallucination commonly implies, or can they refer to a different
kind of reality? This is not the proper place to discuss this
epistemological question. But for an authoritative treatment of
the problem, I refer you to Joseph Maréchal's remarkable

27. Picot de Clorivière, *Considérations sur l'exercise de la prière* (1802), quoted in A.
Poulain, *The Graces of Interior Prayer* (St. Louis, Mo.: Herder, 1910), p. 78. Why so
much special attention is given to memory will appear further along in this paper.

28. Scaramelli, in his renowned *Directorio mistico* (1754: Treatise 3, #32), does not
hesitate to use the term *sensation* for those direct perceptions. Luis de la Puente
distinguishes separate senses: "As the body has its exterior senses, with which it
perceives the visible and delectable things of this life, and makes experience of them,
so the spirit with its faculties of understanding and will, has five interior acts
corresponding to these senses, which we call seeing, hearing, smelling, tasting, and
touching spiritually, with which it perceives the invisible and delectable things of
Almighty God, and makes experience of them." *Meditations*, as quoted in Poulain, p.
101.

essay, "On the Feeling of Presence in Mystics and Non-Mystics." [29]

Yet a great deal of caution is required in interpreting references to mystical sensations. What John of the Cross describes as "touches" *(toque)* appears to be totally unrelated to those hallucinatory experiences in which the senses play a direct part and which remain, therefore, subject to errors of interpretation.

> When God himself visits it [the soul] . . . it is in total darkness and in concealment from the enemy that the soul receives these spiritual favors of God. The reason for this is that, as his Majesty dwells substantially in the soul, where neither angel nor devil can attain to an understanding of that which comes to pass, they cannot know the intimate and secret communications which take place there between the soul and God. These communications, since the Lord Himself works them, are wholly divine and sovereign, for they are all substantial touches of Divine union between the soul and God.[30]

Repeatedly John insists that those touches occur "in the substance" of the soul, not in its faculties, and consequently, that they have neither form nor figure.[31] He seems to use the term *touches* to denote an experience unrelated to sensation but analogous to it by its directly intuitive character. The sense of touch was probably selected because of its greater immediacy and lesser distinctness.

As for the imagination, many spiritual writers attribute a new function to it in the visions and voices which usually precede the higher states of union. Imaginary visions may

29. Joseph Maréchal, *Studies in the Psychology of the Mystics*, trans. Algar Thorold (Albany: Magi Books, 1964), pp. 55–146.

30. *Dark Night of the Soul* 2:23, 11. Cf. also 2:23, 5, and *The Living Flame of Love*, trans. E. Allison Peers (New York: Doubleday, 1962), stanza 2, 16, pp. 67–68.

31. *Living Flame of Love*, st. 2, 7, p. 62.

appear with the intensity of actual sensations yet without any
hallucinatory sensory experiences, and often in fantastic or
unprecedented forms.[32] It is as if images and symbols normally
restricted to the unconscious were released when the mind first
penetrates into the unknown depths of itself.[33] Jung has
written memorable pages on this release of unconscious types
and symbols.[34] The mystical vision structures this "unconscious" material according to its own intentionality. It would
therefore be mistaken to place those visions on a par with
ordinary dreams, in which the same or similar material may appear. Indeed, St. Teresa points out that the imaginary vision
is often accompanied by an "intellectual" one which it renders
more vivid and to which it gives a more lasting impact.[35]

Nevertheless, the upper levels of the unconscious appear to
be more autonomous here than at any other stage of the
mystical experience. Spiritual directors almost universally
adopt a critical attitude toward this most sensational aspect of
the mystical life. Zen masters as well as Christian directors
caution the novice not to attach any importance to those
apparitions.[36] Even if they come from God, St. John of the

32. Teresa describes the imaginary vision as being "so clear that it seems like
reality" and "a living image" which the imagination is unable to produce in its
ordinary functioning. "How could we picture Christ's Humanity by merely studying
the subject or form any impression of His great beauty by means of the imagination?"
The Autobiography of St. Teresa of Avila, trans. and ed. E. Allison Peers (New York:
Doubleday, 1960), pp. 268, 261, 262.

33. In writing *first* I do not wish to imply that those states are restricted to one
particular stage of development. They may be part of a recurring experience, as they
clearly were in St. Teresa's case.

34. *Psychology and Religion: West and East*, trans. R. F. C. Hull (London, 1958), pp.
542–52. Jung's interpretation was vaguely anticipated by William James, *The Varieties
of Religious Experience* (New York: Collier Books, 1961), p. 375, and, uncritically, by H.
Delacroix, *Etudes sur l'histoire et la psychologie des grands mystiques chrétiens* (Paris, 1908).

35. "Though the former type of vision [the intellectual], which, as I said, reveals
God without presenting any image of Him, is of a higher kind, yet, if the memory of it
is to last . . . it is a great thing that so divine a Presence should be presented to the
imagination and should remain within it. These two kinds of vision almost invariably
occur simultaneously." *The Autobiography of St. Teresa of Avila*, p. 263.

36. William Johnston, explaining the suspicion with which the phenomena of the

Cross warns us, they are "curtains and veils covering the
spiritual thing." [37] True spiritual communication takes place
on a deeper level, and all attention spent on those intermediate phenomena detracts from the direct contemplation of what
remains beyond perception and imagination. Nevertheless, St.
John attempts to justify the existence of those imaginary
visions and, in doing so, approaches a modern, psychological
interpretation of the phenomenon.

> If God is to move the soul and to raise it up from the
> extreme depth of its lowliness to the extreme height of His
> loftiness, in Divine union with Him, He must do it with
> order and sweetness and according to the nature of the
> soul itself. Then, since the order whereby the soul
> acquires knowledge is through forms and images of
> created things, and the natural way wherein it acquires
> this knowledge and wisdom is through the senses, it
> follows that, if God is to raise up the soul to supreme
> knowledge, and to do so with sweetness, He must begin to
> work from the lowest and extreme end of the senses of the
> soul, in order that He may gradually lead it, according to
> its own nature, to the other extreme of His spiritual
> wisdom, which belongs not to sense. [38]

A further discussion of those states belongs to the psychology of
mysticism. Our present purpose is merely to explore what the
mystical experience contributes to the knowledge of the self as
such. From that point of view the highest states of mysticism,

---

"makyo" stage in the developing Zen enlightenment are regarded, interprets it as the
rising of the unconscious into the conscious mind (*The Still Point*, pp. 10, 50). St. John
of the Cross claims that "both God and the devil can represent the same images and
species." *The Ascent of Mount Carmel*, trans. and ed. E. Allison Peers (New York:
Doubleday, 1958), 2:16, 3. Even Teresa, who reports some of her most striking visions
as having been of this kind, nevertheless adds that they are open to "illusions of the
devil," and that she herself has been deceived by them. *Autobiography*, chap. 28, esp.
pp. 259, 263.

37. *Ascent of Mount Carmel* 2:16, 11; also 2:19.
38. Ibid., 2:17, 3.

in which the so-called intellectual visions take place, are the most important ones, because they are totally unique and incomparable to any other experiences.

First it must be emphasized that there is more to those states than visions, even though we shall concentrate on them for practical reasons. Next, "intellectual visions" are not visions proper, since they do not consist of perceptions or images. Nor are they "intellectual" in the ordinary sense, since they are entirely nondiscursive and contribute nothing to the subject's "understanding" of himself and his world. Nevertheless, their main impact is one of insight, and even of all-surpassing insight. Since the reader may not be familiar with descriptions of this kind of experience, I here relate two clear instances of it taken from Teresa and Ignatius of loyola. Teresa writes:

> I once had such great light from the presence of the Three Persons which I bear in my soul that it was impossible for me to doubt that the true and living God was present, and I then came to understand things which I shall never be able to describe. One of these was how human flesh was taken by the Person of the Son and not by the other Persons. As I say, I shall never be able to explain any of this, for there are some things which take place in such secret depths of the soul that the understanding seems to comprehend them only like a person who, though sleeping or half asleep, believes he is understanding what is being told him.[39]

Even more typical is Ignatius' description of what he experienced at the river Cardoner:

> As he sat there, the eyes of his understanding began to open. Without having any vision he understood—knew—many matters both spiritual and pertaining to the Faith

39. *Relations*, in *Works*, trans. E. Allison Peers (London, 1934–35), 1:362.

and the realm of letters and that with such clearness that they seemed utterly new to him. There is no possibility of setting out in detail everything he then understood. The most that he can say is that he was given so great an enlightening of his mind that if one were to put together all the helps he has received from God and all the things he has ever learned, they would not be the equal of what he received in that single illumination. He was left with his understanding so enlightened that he seemed to be another man with another mind than the one that was his before.[40]

The only mystic who has attempted to explain those experiences is John of the Cross. If I understand his interpretation correctly, the purely intellectual "apprehensions" may still have a certain sensory orientation, in the sense that some affect the subject as visions would affect him, others as voices, and still others as touches, yet always "without any kind of apprehension concerning form, images or figure of natural fancy or imagination." [41] If this is the case, then Teresa's words make sense when she writes that "the Lord Himself in an *intellectual vision so clear that it seemed almost imaginary,* laid Himself in my arms." [42]

Still, for our purpose it may be more profitable to concentrate on the purely spiritual content. All visions of this nature are short, ecstatic, and, in spite of their abundant spiritual light, somewhat obscure. Among the visions of incorporeal substances, St. John of the Cross mentions a direct vision of the soul. He also claims that the intellectual experiences are "felt in the substance of the soul." [43] "God works then in the soul

40. *Obras Completas de san Ignacio de Loyola,* trans. Elmer O'Brien (Madrid, 1952), pp. 49–50, in *Varieties of Mystic Experience,* p. 247.
41. *Ascent of Mount Carmel,* 2:23, 3.
42. *Relations, Works* 1:364.
43. *Ascent of Mount Carmel,* 2:24, 4, and 24, 2.

without making use of its own capacities." [44] From all
evidence, we confront here unified states of consciousness
which allow the soul to contact its own core. Let us subject this
metaphorical language to a critical analysis.

The Substance of the Soul

First, even those unified states of consciousness retain a
noetic quality which allows the mystics to refer to them as
intellectual.[45] Yet the mind escapes the duality of ordinary
consciousness. Taken literally, the expression "beyond dreamless sleep" in the *Mandukya Upanishad* would place the highest
mystical state outside consciousness altogether. Yet the *Brhad-
Aranyaka* explains, "Verily while he does not think, he is verily
thinking." [46] However, the thought is not a second thing
separate from the thinker. This is indicated by John's claim
that intellectual visions take place "in the substance of the
soul," and by the various other expressions referring to
substance at the end of *The Dark Night*, such as "His Majesty
dwells substantially in the soul" and "substantial touches of
Divine union between the soul and God." [47] Clearly, the term
substance alone appeared appropriate for that coincidence of
being and knowing which precedes all mental differentiation.

Whatever else this knowledge may contain, it includes a
unique and direct awareness of the self. Its direct character is
all the more remarkable, since it is described entirely in
negative terms. One attentive reader of the Christian mystics
writes:

44. Ibid., 26, 5.

45. William James was undoubtedly right in ascribing this quality to all mystical
states. Cf. *Varieties of Religious Experience*, p. 300.

46. *Brhad-Aranyaka*, 4, 3, 28, in Hume, *Thirteen Principal Upanishads*. Teresa, in a text
which strongly emphasizes the total passivity of the experience, qualifies her assertion
about the lack of knowledge: "Here we are all asleep, and fast asleep to the things of
the world, and to ourselves." *Interior Castle* (Fifth Mansions), trans. E. Allison Peers
(New York: Doubleday, 1961), p. 97.

47. *Dark Night of the Soul*, 2:23, 11.

The soul empties itself absolutely of every specific operation and of all multiplicity, and knows negatively by
means of the void and the annihilation of every act and of
every object of thought coming from outside—the soul
knows negatively—but nakedly, without veils—that metaphysical marvel, that absolute, that perfection of every
act and of every perfection, which is *to exist,* which is the
soul's own substantial existence.[48]

Whether the right term is *existence,* as Maritain claims, or
essence, as it is called by many mystics, all agree that we have
here a direct—although negative—knowledge of ultimate
selfhood, an immediate awareness of presence to oneself and to
the transcendent source of the self. Such a direct intuition
bypasses the channels of sensation and judgment by which the
awareness of the self is usually attained. It neither needs nor
provides any rational justification of itself. Confronted with
statements such as "I felt that God was there: I saw Him
neither with my bodily eyes nor through my imagination,
nevertheless His presence was certain to me," [49] it is difficult
not to accept the existence of a direct mental intuition in the
mystical state. Most epistemologists have followed Kant in
denying that the human mind ever attains such a *direct* insight
into the presence of the real as such. Yet even Kantian
students of the mystical experience are forced to admit that no
other explanation remains.[50] For this fully conscious being-

48. Jacques Maritain, *Redeeming the Time* (London: Geoffrey Bles, 1946), p. 242.
Maritain distinguishes between the "natural" mystical experience, in which the soul is
attained directly and God indirectly; and the "supernatural," in which God is
attained directly (p. 246). I am not sure that such a distinction can be consistently
maintained on a theological level, much less on a philosophical one. In all religious
mysticism the self is immediately perceived *in* its transcendent dimension or, in
Maritain's language, in its "sources."

49. Luis de la Puente, *Vida del P. Balthasar Alvarez* (Madrid, 1615), chap. 15; trans.
and quoted in Poulain, *Graces of Interior Prayer,* p. 83.

50. This is especially the case for Joseph Maréchal (cf. *Psychology of the Mystics,* pp.
102, 196). But we find it also in Rudolf Otto, *Mysticism East and West,* trans. Bertha L.

with-oneself cannot be accounted for by the categories of ordinary consciousness. The ordinary awareness of the self is achieved indirectly through a reflection upon its operations. Yet in mystical states we attain a direct, explicit awareness of the self *as such.*

> And this knowledge shows itself so radically different from ordinary knowledge, from the threefold standpoint of immediateness, mode and content, that the contemplative remains in the deepest stupefaction thereat. For in this case it is not amnesia which appears after the ecstasy any more than it was complete unconsciousness during it; the mystic remembers perfectly, but he does it through the belittling and dividing forms of the understanding which once more oppress him.[51]

Those words of Maréchal's echo John of the Cross's conclusion: "It is like one who sees something never seen before, whereof he has not even seen the like. . . . How much less, then, could he describe a thing that has not entered through the senses." [52]

Some of the insight into the self acquired through mystical experience was thematized in various developments of Augustine's theory of memory. In *De Trinitate XIV*, 13, 17, memory is said to contain the mind's latent knowledge of itself and of God. By wisdom *(sapientia)* "distinct from knowledge, conferred by God's gift through a partaking in God himself," [53] the mind *recognizes* what it knew implicitly. The knowledge of God here coincides with the ultimate knowledge of the self.

Bracey and Richenda C. Payne (New York: Macmillan, 1932 [1970]), pp. 50–88, and, with some qualifications, in the Thomist Jacques Maritain, *Distinguish to Unite*, trans. Gerald Phelan (New York: Scribner's, 1959), pp. 261 ff. and 446–50. Compare with St. Thomas, *Summa Theologiae* II–II 180, 5.

51. Maréchal, p. 192.
52. *Dark Night of the Soul*, 2:17, 3.
53. *De Trinitate XV*, 3, 5.

Even in Augustine this theory is more than a Christian adaptation of Plato's theory of *anamnesis,* because the religious experience in Augustine always precedes the categories, borrowed or invented, in which he expresses it. Mystical writers will adopt this theory of memory and develop its Trinitarian aspect. Thus, for William of St. Thierry, just as the Father is the silent source of the Word, so memory is the silent ground of the soul from which the work of cognition proceeds.[54] This theory is developed more systematically by the Franciscans Alexander of Hales and Bonaventure. In the third chapter of his *Itinerarium Mentis ad Deum,* Bonaventure concludes:

> And thus through the operation of the memory, it appears that the soul itself is the image of God and His likeness, so present to itself and having Him present that it receives Him in actuality and is susceptible of receiving Him in potency, and that it can also participate in Him.[55]

In the Vedantic tradition the mystical knowledge of a self that remains hidden from ordinary awareness is all the more emphasized since the duality between man and Brahman is abolished. This fundamental self, unknowable yet attainable, is the ultimate reality. Shankara built his entire mystical philosophy on it. The "ground" of the soul, the Atman beyond all functions of consciousness, is the locus of mystical truth. This ground of selfhood is experienced by the mystics not only as hidden but also as transcendent. It is the very point in which the soul is more than an individual soul. Thus, in the Vedantic tradition this deeper self is at once the core of all that is:

> The Inner Soul of all things, the One Controller,
> Who makes his one form manifold—

---

54. William of St. Thierry; cf. "The Trinitarian Ascent of the Soul to God in the Theology of William of St. Thierry," *Recherches de théologie ancienne et médiévale* 26 (1959): 85–127.

55. *The Mind's Road to God,* trans. George Boas (Indianapolis: Bobbs-Merrill, 1953), p. 23.

The wise who perceive Him as standing in oneself,
They, and no others, have eternal happiness.[56]

Now, he who on all beings
Looks as just in the Self,
And on the Self as in all beings—
He does not shrink away from Him.[57]

Texts such as the preceding one clearly indicate that the ground of the self far surpasses the boundaries of individual personhood.

Christians tend to write this off as oriental pantheism. But upon careful scrutiny they will find that their own mystics assert the transcendence of the mystical self. To them also at one point the soul and God are not two but one. We recall Eckhart's daring language: "There is something in the soul so closely akin to God that it is already one with Him and need never be united to Him. . . . If one were wholly this, he would be both uncreated and unlike any creature." [58] Most Christian mystics have been less radical in their expression but not in their meaning. Thus Johann Tauler refers to the soul as a creature, but one standing between eternity and time, and with its supernatural part entirely in eternity.[59]

Yet no one has elaborated the theme of self-transcendence more consistently and with more theological strength than Jan Ruusbroec. According to the Flemish mystic, man's true essence (wesen) is his superessence (overwesen). Before its creation the soul is present in God as a pure image: this divine image remains its superessence after its actual creation.[60] The mystical conversion, then, consists for Ruusbroec in regaining

---

56. *Katha Upanishad* 5, 12, Hume, *Thirteen Principal Upanishads*, p. 357.

57. *Isa Upanishad* 6, Hume, p. 363.

58. Sermon "Qui audit me, non confundetur," in *Meister Eckhart*, p. 205.

59. "Sermon for Christmas," in *Signposts to Perfection*, pp. 3–4.

60. *Een Spieghel der Eeuwigher Salicheit*, in Jan Van Ruusbroec, *Werken* (Tielt: Lannoo, 1947), 3:167.

mystical conversion, then, consists for Ruusbroec in regaining one's uncreated image. Through the mystical transformation (which Ruusbroec calls "over-formation"), the soul surpasses its createdness and participates actively in God's uncreated life.

> All those men who are raised up above their created being into a contemplative life are one with this divine brightness and are that brightness itself. And they see, feel and find, even by means of this Divine Light, that, as regards their uncreated nature, they are that same simple ground from which the brightness without limit shines forth in a godlike manner, and which according to the simplicity of the essence remains in everlasting, mode-less simplicity.[61]

To Ruusbroec, the soul is from all eternity an archetype within God. To the extent that its actual existence in time is essentially connected with this archetypal image, it "dwells in God, flows forth from God, depends upon God and returns to God." [62] The nobleness which the mind possesses by its very nature, it cannot lose without ceasing to exist altogether. Now free, created mind may *actualize* the dynamic tendency of its nature "toward the Image" through a virtuous and God-seeking life. Yet a total identification can occur only through the passive graces of the "God-seeing" life. In the mystical state, the mind comes to live "above nature" "in the essential unity of God's own being, at the summit of his spirit." [63]

Thus the ultimate message of the mystic about the nature of selfhood is that the self is *essentially* more than a mere self, that transcendence belongs to its nature as much as the act through which it is immanent to itself, and that a total failure on the

61. *Die gheestelike brulocht*, in *Werken* 1:246. *The Adornment of Spiritual Marriage*, trans. C. A. Wynschenck (New York: E. P. Dutton, 1916), p. 174.

62. *Adornment of Spiritual Marriage*, p. 127.

63. Ibid., p. 130.

mind's part to realize this transcendence reduces the self to *less* than itself. It is in this dynamic view of a potentially unlimited mind that I find the most significant contribution to a philosophical understanding of the self.

6

The Existential Approach to Psychiatry*

ERWIN W. STRAUS

In September of 1958 psychotherapists from many countries convened at an international congress in Barcelona, Spain. The central topic of that meeting was existential analysis and psychotherapy. Existential analysis—the English equivalent of the German term *Daseinsanalyse*—is to a great extent the work of one man, Ludwig Binswanger, a Swiss psychiatrist. He made it his task to apply the ontology of the philosopher Martin Heidegger to psychiatry, turning Heidegger's *Analytic of Dasein*—a word that occurs in the singular only—into *Daseinsanalysen*, existential analyses, practically unlimited in number. Heidegger, Binswanger's philosophical master, was one of the many pupils of Edmund Husserl (1859–1938). In 1900, the same year in which Freud published his *Interpretation of Dreams*, Husserl presented his *Logical Investigations*, his primer on the way to phenomenology. Existential therapy in psychiatry, therefore, is the fourth in a line of descent which leads from phenomenology to philosophy of existence, from philosophy of existence to existential analysis, and from existential analysis to existential therapy.

Husserl's influence on continental thinking is still growing or, one could say, is growing anew through the posthumous editions of his later works, unpublished—partly for political

---

* Presented at the Unitarian Symposium on Man's Inner World, The Resources of Religion and Depth Psychology, Cincinnati, Ohio, Feb. 19, 1960.

reasons—at the time of the philosopher's death. As so often happens in situations like this, there are pupils who faithfully adhere to the doctrines of their teacher and others who depart from the orthodox line. Heidegger is one of the outstanding heretics. There are many branches of phenomenology today, but there would be no phenomenology at all without Husserl. It will be my task here to condense years of the history of ideas into a brief essay.

If I had to select the one concept most characteristic for phenomenology, comparable to the role ascribed to the unconscious in psychoanalysis, I would choose the term *intentionality*. Intentionality of consciousness—most phenomenologists would agree—is the central theme of phenomenology. The term *intentionality* registers the fact that every act of consciousness is directed to an object, that perception is a perception of something remembered, a remembering of something, etc. This statement certainly sounds trivial; one might wonder how such a truism could justify the claim of signifying a new style in philosophy.

The answer to this objection is that modern science, since its beginning in the seventeenth century, has more and more discarded everyday life experience. In the course of centuries the very foundations of human experience and knowledge have been screened from sight by the theoretical structures erected upon them. Intentionality of consciousness, therefore, was discovered—or to put it more accurately, was rediscovered—by Brentano in the field of empirical psychology before Husserl put the natural position in question and proceeded to the distinction of the empirical from the transcendental ego. Phenomenology is—at least in one respect—a critique of the unconditional application of physics to human existence. It challenges the positivist claim of the universal validity of natural science. The physicist may take the possibility of observing, measuring, predicting, for granted. However, in the humane sciences man plays a double role: he is the observed but also the observer. The genuine themes of psychology, therefore, are the seeing of visible things, the measuring of observable objects, the predicting of things to come.

Phenomenology considers physics as a human creation, rooted in the experience of everyday life—the intersubjective experience of our world in its macroscopic structure and the fullness of sensory qualities. The scientist, with all his procedures of observing and measuring, with all the instruments at his disposal, never leaves our common, everyday-life world. Phenomenology inquires into the basic structure of the everyday-life world which makes scientific behavior possible as one of the many forms of the human enterprise. In short, phenomenology strictly contradicts the tenets of scientific empiricism, which holds "that only physical phenomena are the material with which psychology, like any other natural science, is concerned." The behavioral sciences obviously tend to apply the principles of physics to the physicist himself; they assume that there is no realm of reality inaccessible to the methods of the natural sciences.

This assumption is nothing new; it is based on metaphysical speculations, centuries old. Yet very few know their family tree more than three or four generations back. Still less known is the ancestry of our basic scientific postulates. Let us, then, start now on a kind of cinerama tour through the first centuries of modern science.

The founding fathers of modern science (Galileo, Descartes, Hobbes) were decided revolutionaries. Their revolt was directed against the "schools"—namely, against scholasticism, that blend of Christian theology and Greek philosophy, and against the authority of the Bible. Enchanted by the freedom of thinking and by the power promised through the technical application of their discoveries, they inadvertently undermined man's position in the universe. Modern man, triumphant in his conquest of nature, today desperately searches for any meaning in his existence.

"The world which Science presents for our belief," wrote Bertrand Russell in 1902,

> is . . . purposeless, void of meaning. . . . That Man is the product of causes which had no prevision of the end they were achieving; that his origin, his growth, his hopes and fears, his loves and his beliefs, are but the outcome of accidental collocations of atoms; that no fire, no heroism, no intensity of thought and feeling, can preserve an individual life beyond the grave; that all the labours of the ages, all the devotion, all the inspiration, all the noonday brightness of human genius, are destined to extinction in the vast death of the solar system, and that the whole temple of Man's achievement must inevitably be buried beneath the debris of a universe in ruins—all these things, if not quite beyond dispute, are yet so nearly certain, that no philosophy which rejects them can hope to stand. . . . Blind to good and evil, reckless of destruction, omnipotent matter rolls on its relentless way; for Man, condemned to-day to lose his dearest, to-morrow himself to pass through the gate of darkness, it remains only to cherish, ere yet the blow falls, the lofty thoughts that ennoble his little day; disdaining the coward terrors of the slave of Fate, to worship at the shrine that his own hands have built; undismayed by the empire of chance, to preserve a mind free from the wanton tyranny that rules his outward life; proudly defiant of the irresistible forces that tolerate, for a moment, his knowledge and his condemnation, to sustain alone, a weary but unyielding Atlas, the world that his own ideals have fashioned despite the trampling march of unconscious power.[1]

Measurement, experiments, and the application of mathe-

---

1. Bertrand Russell, "A Free Man's Worship," in *Mysticism and Logic, and Other Essays* (Penguin Books, 1953), pp. 51, 59.

matics are often claimed as the significant traits of modern science. Yet the names of Archimedes and Ptolemy remind us that measurement, experiments, and the application of mathematics were not alien to the Greek scientists and astronomers. However, in their philosophy of nature, the universe was conceived as a cosmos, as one finite, beautifully ordered whole. Such a well-ordered whole needs to be divided into different regions. In Aristotle's cosmology, accepted by scholastic philosophers, space was not considered homogeneous as it was later, in Galilean and Newtonian physics. Things had their natural places where they would come to rest. No uniform type of mathematics was applicable to the universe as a whole.

In this pre-Copernican cosmology, the earth, as everybody knows, occupied a central position. The geocentric orientation did not mean that the earth was considered more noble than the stars. In fact, in traditional evaluation the sublunar world appeared less divine than the stars moving in their perfect order. Nevertheless, man was placed above all other creatures because he was endowed with speech and reason: in Aristotle's definition, an animal that has logos—Man, the rational animal—was believed to be able to comprehend the world, rational in its own structure.

Galileo (1564–1642) shared this conviction of rationality with the philosophers of antiquity. He thought that nature was a book written in mathematical terms; God had created the world as a geometrician, and the human mind could figure out the geometric structures of the universe. Although the application of mathematics was then nothing new, the style of mathematics itself had undergone a transformation between the time of Euclid and the time of Galileo. The transition from the geocentric to the heliocentric system was perhaps not as radical a change as the new idea of a world extended into an infinite homogeneous space.

Copernicus, Galileo, and Kepler might not have been successful had not Luther and Calvin prepared the transformation of cosmological views. Down to the age of the Reformation, God, in the religious feeling of Western mankind, was close to our world. He was omnipotent; his presence was most strongly felt in the liturgy of the mass. But the Reformation established an unsurmountable distance between the creation and the creator. God was conceived of as *deus absconditus,* and thereby the world was abandoned by God. Descartes did not hesitate to exploit the situation opened by the theologians. In an ironical reversal of the biblical story of man's expulsion from paradise, modern science denied to the creator reentrance into his own creation. Interference with the mechanisms of the universe was not reconcilable with God's majesty, Descartes taught, because in any case He would have changed matters from a perfect to a less perfect condition. Indeed, the basic laws of conservation of energy (conceived first by Descartes as conservation of the total amount of motion) demanded His noninterference; at this point physics and theology were most intimately interwoven. In seventeenth-century writings God is frequently likened unto a watchmaker who made the universe like a watch and set it in motion. We can find out the structure of this clockwork, which in its astronomical dimensions includes man himself as just another little wheel in the machinery. The same laws of nature regulate the macrocosmos and the human microcosmos.

Galileo made the most impressive beginning in analyzing the mechanics of the universe. With the expectation that science could ultimately solve all the riddles of human existence, science was to be established as the knowledge of exact, immutable, quantifiable relations expressed in mathematical equations. However, in our observation of nature things do not comply with these requirements. They appear in a perspective of ever-changing conditions of light and darkness; they are colorful, red or green, and hot or cold, rough or smooth. The sensory qualities would not yield to mathematical treatment. Galileo solved the problem presented by their resistance through a coup de force. He declared that colors and sounds are not real; they exist only in our minds.

> As soon as I conceive a piece of material I feel myself impelled of conceiving that in its own nature it is bounded and figured in such and such a figure, that in relation to others it is large or small, that it is in this or that place, in this or that time, that it is in motion or remains at rest, that it touches or does not touch another body, that it is single, few, or many; . . . but that it must be white or red, bitter or sweet, sounding or mute, of a pleasant or unpleasant odour, I do not perceive my mind forced to acknowledge. . . . Hence I think that these tastes, odours, colours, etc., on the side of the object in which they seem to exist, are nothing else than mere names, but hold their residence solely in the sensitive body; so that if the animal were removed, every such quality would be abolished and annihilated.[2]

This distinction of shape, size, number, motion, and rest, from colors, sounds, heat, etc., as primary and secondary qualities (John Locke invented the terminology) was eminently useful for physics but likewise fateful for the human sciences. If color and heat were not true "affections and qualities really residing in the thing we perceive," [3] the physicist was no longer committed to account for them. But the metaphysical devaluation did not annihilate secondary qualities; they continued to exist. After all, man's environment and stage of action is one of secondary qualities. What could it mean to say that colors and heat reside in our minds? Must one assume different levels of reality: one objective or truly

2. Galileo, *Il Saggiatore, Opere complete*, 4:333 ff.; see E. A. Burtt, *The Metaphysical Foundations of Modern Science* (New York: Anchor Books, 1954), p. 85.
3. Burtt, *Metaphysical Foundations*.

real and the other one merely subjective and illusionary? If colors and sounds are subjective, must this not hold true for brightness, and finally for the geometric patterns also? Is it scientifically justifiable to perform the physicalistic reduction and continue to talk about us and our minds? If colors are relative to man, is not man relative to a world of colors and sounds?

René Descartes's *Metaphysics* provided an answer to at least some of the problems linked with the Galilean doctrine of subjectivism. According to Descartes, there are two regions of reality: a field of an extended substance *(res extensa)*; and the realm of a thinking substance *(res cogitans),* identified also with mind, soul, consciousness. The two substances, although radically different, are of equal ontological rank. Colors and sounds, considered solely as data of consciousness, are no less real than figure and size. Unfortunately, we, succumbing to a habit acquired in early childhood, fall prey to the error of treating them as if they were objective attributes of physical things. Descartes's distinction between two substances, with the ensuing dichotomy of mind and body, placed consciousness into exile outside nature; consciousness appeared extramundane. Since the time of Descartes, one speaks about an external world to which we have no direct access. Yet, in spite of the radical separation of mind from body, Descartes also claimed that in man—and in man only—the two substances were united. For obvious reasons he was unable to explain how such a unification could ever occur. Generations of philosophers have labored to solve this riddle.

Still, I must mention one of them, because the solution proposed by him continues to dominate the thinking of many scientists in our day. Thomas Hobbes rejected Descartes's metaphysical dualism only to preserve it in a modified form. According to Hobbes, only one of the two substances, the *res extensa,* is real.

> For light and colour, and heat and sound, and other qualities which are commonly called sensible, are in the

object which causeth them but so many several motions of
the matter, by which it presseth our organs diversely.
Neither in us that are pressed are they any thing else but
diverse motions (for motion produceth nothing but motion). But their appearance to us is Fancy, the same
waking that dreaming.[4]

The scientist therefore has to relate these phantasmas to the
underlying neuromechanisms.

Hobbes turned the distinction of primary and secondary
quantities, as you see, upon man himself. In its original form it
was related and restricted to physical bodies. The primary
quantities were considered objective, and the secondary purely
subjective. Our mathematical perceptions and ideas supposedly are in correspondence with the real configuration of
physical bodies; our sensory experience in its totality is
secondary, for all data of consciousness are derived from the
senses and share with them the metaphysical devaluation to
mere phantasmas and images. Consciousness, therefore, could
not add anything to neural events; it could not expand the
reach of experiencing beings beyond the here and now; it does
not open the world to us; it does not establish a relation to
objects qua objects.

Let me illustrate the situation through an example. In
everyday life we are convinced that the driver of a car is aware
of his environment and of his own position in relation to street,
trees, pedestrians, and other vehicles. From his egocentric
position he drives toward a goal. Scientific interpretation
denies that these relations deserve serious consideration. It
explains the behavior—for instance, of a driver—as the result
of synaptic connections acquired in the past through conditioning. The epiphenomenalistic theory replaces meaningful
conduct with functions of mechanisms deprived of meaning; it
supplants the I-world relation with events within a body.

4. Thomas Hobbes, *Leviathan*, bk. 1, chap. 1.

This whole process of reduction is performed in perplexing naïveté! The behaviorist never considers his own behavior and activities; he stubbornly ignores the fact that the stimulus-response schema must be applicable to himself; it must be equally valid for the observer. Two brains are involved in all neurophysiological and psychological experiments: the brain observed and the brain of the observer. In everyday-life parlance we may say that an observer sees an object; translated into scientific language, we must say that an observer's receptors were activated by optical stimuli. Observation must be reduced to afferent and efferent impulses located in the observer's nervous system. Obviously the stimulus-response schema leaves no room for awareness of any object qua object. How then is science—how is observing, describing, measuring—possible? The answer requires one to realize and to acknowledge the chasm separating the relation of an experiencing being to an object, from the relation of a nervous system to a stimulus. At this point the concept of the "intentionality of consciousness" manifests its truth and fruitfulness.

Although my eyes are affected by the light reflected from this paper before me, I nevertheless see it as the other, something existing independent from me. In fact, one could perhaps define consciousness as that condition which makes it possible that one part in this world of ours is related to another one, as to the other. Those, from Ecclesiastes to Bertrand Russell, who reminded us that man is nothing but a speck of dust were inclined to overlook the fact that this mote can conceive the whole of the universe to which it belongs as a part. The reach of experiencing beings, men and animals, extends beyond their here-and-now.

In my own work I have tried to "save" sensory experience from theoretical misinterpretations and then to apply the regained understanding of the norm to pathological manifestations.

In sensory experience everyone is at the center of his world, opened to him within a temporo-spatial horizon as a zone of possible action. When I walk toward that chair over there, I am moving at this moment toward a potential goal in the future, although some photic rays have already stimulated my retina. In this primary egocentric position we experience the world in relation to us as appealing or repelling. Sensory experience is first of all in the service of self-preservation; it orients the individual as a living organism in relation to objects desirable or rejectable. Our primary relation to the world is not that of an "objective" scientific observer. To us as mortal creatures, supported but also threatened by the environment, things appear in physiognomic aspects. Man is able to detach himself from the original relationship and learn to see objects in their own context and framework.

Traditionally, sense perception is interpreted as the presence of an image produced by a stimulating object in the recipient's brain or mind. In everyday life we realize that we see something with our own eyes, that in looking at a hot stove and in touching it we are affected in different ways. In short, in sensory experience we are aware of an object *and* of ourselves. We experience our very existence in relation to the other. Were it not so, we could never apprehend an object as an object. In sensory perception, we are never the neutral onlooker; we are personally involved, seized in a certain manner, according to the characteristics of each sense modality. Reality is experienced immediately, as a coexistence of the world and myself. In the realm of sensory experience, *real* means something happens to me, while in a scientific attitude the predicate *real* indicates that something occurs in agreement with the established laws of nature. In the first case, reality is sensed in a personal relation to me or you; in the second, it is the tenet of an impersonal proposition.

This distinction between personal, egocentric sensory experience and detached perception and observation is of paramount importance for psychiatry, for it opens an avenue to the understanding of some of the most impressive psychotic symptoms. Hallucinations and delusions, for instance, occur on the level of immediate experience. Because the patient is overwhelmed by the power of sensory experience, hallucinations and delusions will not yield to any critical argumentation. The I-world relationship is the basic structure of both normal and pathological experience.

The term "I-world relation" certainly resembles Heidegger's title "Being-in-the-world" as the first characteristic of human existence. In spite of this resemblance, however, there are important differences. Heidegger's central theme is a quest for the meaning of Being. Being, spelled with a capital *B*, corresponds to the German infinitive noun *das Sein*, the Latin *esse*, and the French *être*. Heidegger's book *Being and Time*[5] is an ontological study, concerned with Being—not with beings, which constitute the topic of the positive sciences. This ontic ontological difference must be clearly understood; in reading and reporting Heidegger one must never lose sight of this distinction. His interpretation of human life is put in the service of that main ontological purpose; *Analytic of Dasein* is a means toward the end of comprehending the meaning of Being.

Why can an interpretation of human life serve that purpose better than the traditional analysis of "nature" and physical events? Heidegger's answer is that man is distinguished from all other living creatures by the fact that "he always relates himself to his own Being. In some way he always understands his Being, and he is always concerned about his Being and the possibilities of his Being." Concerned with the possibilities of his Being, he steps out in his projects from the actual present toward the future. Taking the Latin word *existere* literally—as *ex-istere*—Heidegger used it to signify just this mode of

5. Martin Heidegger, *Sein und Zeit* (Fed. Tübingen: Niemeyer, 1953).

transcending. The term *existence* in Heidegger's first period of production signifies that man always transcends the boundaries of the here and now toward his own possibilities. There is an open horizon of the unique and undetermined surrounding human existence. Therefore, man cannot be comprehended by the usual concepts of essences—that is to say, as a specimen of the species homo sapiens. For this reason Heidegger avoids the term *man* or *human being* but instead speaks of *Dasein*.

Until Heidegger's day, this word was used as a rather harmless vocable of the German language. One spoke about human or animal *Dasein* much in line with the meaning of human or animal existence. Heidegger attached to the vernacular word a new connotation fitting his interpretation of man from the point of view of existence. But the connotation of the term *existence*—as already indicated—also had to be changed. It no longer had the trivial meaning of "there is something," or "something occurs," but referred to the specific and human possibility of transcending oneself.

In the first section of *Analytic of Dasein*, Heidegger considers man in his workshop, if I may say so. Just as the biblical Adam was created as a man fully grown, so *Dasein*, the new Adam, appears without infancy. Heidegger visits man in his house, surrounded by utensils. The possibility of the production of the human environment is not discussed, an omission justified—perhaps—through Heidegger's insistence that in his mode of Being man is radically different from all animals.

At many points in these and later chapters the word *Dasein* displays a power of its own. There are statements that one can make in relation to *Dasein* but not in relation to man; and there are other statements one cannot make about *Dasein* which are indispensable in an anthropology. For example, one can say "*Dasein* is always my own" but could not say "man is always my own." On the other hand, while man is born either male or female, the gender of *Dasein* is neutral. The pronoun *it* refers to *Dasein*. Because we are born men or women, no single individual can be representative for the genus man. By nature everyone is incomplete but capable of and in need of completion by the other one. This natural situation—although not omitted—plays no significant role in Heidegger's anthropological interpretation.

The term *Dasein,* as such, also proves very useful in the second part of analytics, which deals with the "who" of *Dasein.* "*Dasein* is being-with," Heidegger emphasizes. This ontological characteristic eliminates the thorny problem of the alter ego. It also makes it clear that as a rule we are lost in the "faceless crowd." Everyone is inclined to act as one acts, to talk as one talks. Everyone behaves as one of the many. In this type of "unauthentic" existence I do not act as I could or should as a truly unique individual. We all fall prey to unauthenticity, running away from the painful situation of making real choices and irrevocable decisions. Man is thrown into his place. No one has decided for himself to enter into this world. The term *Dasein* also signifies this situation well; *Dasein* is a mode of Being *(Sein)* thrown into its there *(Da)*. *Dasein* responds to its thrownness *(Ge-worfenheit)* with its projects *(Ent-wurf)*. We have to accept our situation and make it our own.

How can one reach authenticity? Heidegger's answer is through facing dread and death—namely, by accepting the nothingness and the finiteness of our existence. At this point Heidegger was no doubt influenced by the Danish philosopher Kierkegaard. Yet Heidegger's position is more radical. Everyone has to reach authenticity in utter loneliness, without help from religion, nature, or society.

In its attempted escape from itself, *Dasein* is held back by the voice of conscience. Existentially, we are always debtors. We always owe something that we should have done but failed to do. (Here Heidegger uses the double connotation of the German word *schulden,* which signifies both owing and being

guilty.) Existential guilt does not mean that we have tres-
passed against certain ethical codes, that we did something not
publicly approved, but that we lived remote from fulfilling the
true possibilities that were ours. At this point the application
of philosophy of existence to psychiatric problems such as
depression, anxiety, and guilt comes into view.

As mentioned in the beginning, it was Ludwig Binswanger
who, several years after the publication of *Being and Time*, tried
to transform Heidegger's *Analytic of Dasein* into *Daseinsanalysen*.
In his case studies, Binswanger investigated *das Dasein* of
individuals, to whom he attached names like Ellen West, Lola
Voss, and others. He studied their particular "thrownness"
and their particular "projects"—in short, their particular
modes of being-in-the-world. Binswanger's existential analysis
—whether a legitimate application of Heidegger's analytic or
not—is by no means a specific psychiatric method. Existential
analysis is not primarily interested in the clinical distinction
between abnormal and normal behavior. In a paper, "The
Human Being in Psychiatry," published in 1956,[6] Binswanger
claims that the psychiatrist cannot be satisfied with looking at
a patient as an object—be it a person, a character, an
organism, or a brain—labeled with a certain clinical diagnosis; the psychiatrist has to approach the patient as a fellow
man in existential communication. Psychotherapy has to be
transformed into an existential encounter—if this should prove
possible.

I have made it my task to report the development which led
from phenomenology to philosophy of existence and existential
analysis and therapy. This historical transition is reflected in
psychiatry as an advance from clinical psychiatry of the

6. Ludwig Binswanger, *Drei Formen missglückten Daseins* (Tübingen: Niemeyer,
1956).

Kraepelinean style to psychoanalysis, and finally to existential analysis. At the turn of the century Kraepelin, Bleuler, and most other psychiatrists considered behavior as a manifestation of the underlying neural mechanism. The norm was identified with the average; psychotic manifestations, all of them supposedly due to organic disturbances, were incomprehensible. Following his studies in hysteria, Freud assumed that psychotic symptoms were meaningful and that the therapist could decipher their coded meaning, tracing them back to their origins. The interpretation of the patient's biographical data became most important.

Yet in these sophisticated chronicles the patient appears as a victim rather than as an agent. In psychoanalysis, the interest of both the therapist and the patient is centered upon the past. In existential analysis the emphasis is on the future. The individual is considered as the actor and author of his projects, who in his choices and decisions succeeds or fails in his self-realization. While Husserl in his thinking and writing was closer to Descartes and Kant than to Hegel and Nietzsche, in Heidegger's work, philosophy of history prevails over philosophy of nature. Being itself is no longer interpreted as unchangeable, lasting, and immutable, but as "pervaded by temporality" and "engendering time" (Zeitigen). Therefore, in the Analytic of Dasein, also, the historical categories—or to be exact, the "existentials"—are dominant. Accordingly, in existential analysis—in contrast to psychoanalysis—the interest is centered on becoming, on the future, and on possibility.

My report leaves many questions unanswered; it may be more appropriate to say it leaves many questions unasked. The information on a "jacket" cannot replace the reading of those books which are demanding without being soothing. This may be one of the reasons why in our day, although we can cross the ocean in six hours, some ideas have required thirty years to make the same passage. I hope that the interest in existential analysis that is flaring up so suddenly will not

fade with the same speed. Perhaps it will be useful to keep in
mind that the chances of survival are better if newcomers are
warned in advance not to look for shortcuts in their studies
and not to expect techniques completely ready for use.

7

Language and the Genealogy
of the Absent Object

JOSEPH H. SMITH

Three familiar passages in Freud that pertain to the absent object are those of the primary model of thought (1900, chap. 7), the *fort-da* game of his grandson (1920, p. 15), and the account of the shadow of the object falling upon the ego, outlined in "Mourning and Melancholia" and developed in *The Ego and the Id*. These may be taken as instances or stages in the genealogy of the absent object.

In the primary model, it is the absence of the object which evokes primitive ideation—the imagery that is the harbinger of language. In the child's game of repeatedly throwing the spool out of sight, then retrieving it, the action and the primitive words designating absence and presence provide a symbolic means of grappling also with the loss of the mother—a loss probably not in the child's awareness during his absorption in the game. In the direct grieving of adults, absence of the object is central in awareness, presiding over the many unconscious processes of internalization by which the work of mourning is accomplished. In *The Ego and the Id*, the significance of internalization is extended to include the mode of development generally; ego and superego development occurs by virtue of the internalization of aspects of lost objects. So, while a genealogy of the absent object explicitly refers to the changing form of the absent object, it implies and runs parallel with the history of the changing form—the develop-ment—of the subject.

In the adult mind, the phrase *absent object* has a primary reference to time past. In the infant, however, there is no such differentiation of the temporal dimensions. Memories are not experienced as memories. Present needs and wishes compel a centrifugal direction and peripheral focus—a reaching out toward the future. This future is molded, to be sure, by the wish into some "likeness of the past," as Freud wrote in that great last sentence of *The Interpretation of Dreams* (1900, p. 621), but not a "perfect likeness" in either primitive or advanced thinking. In the genealogy of the absent object, something of this futural cast of thought going toward its object is main-tained. The line of descent or development is from the absent object, primitively conceived, to clear concepts of certain objects. However, the system of thought and language which allows for clear conceptualization opens up a world wherein any compelling or interesting unknown or unattained assumes the valency and temporal locus of the primitive absent object. Such unknowns are the derivatives of the absent object and continue to evoke thought. Depending on the nature of the person and the nature of the unknown, the approach to the unknown can be primarily in terms of symbolic, or primarily in terms of conceptual, thought. I shall now attempt to define these two modes of approach.

Primary and Secondary Process

To speak of primitive ideation as the harbinger of language is to speak, in psychoanalytic terminology, of the relationship between primary and secondary process. In a rough way, "primary" refers to thinking that is temporally, formally, and topographically earlier or more basic—namely, early in time, more basic in form, and closer to the unconscious. It is unconstrained by the conventions of language, by ordinary rules of logic, by negation, or by temporal dimensions.

Opposites can coexist. The part can represent the whole, and one event or entity can easily represent another or several others. Thinking tends to be in images. It is presumably the dominant mode of thought in infancy. It is clearly the dominant mode in dreaming, in some forms of fantasy and psychosis, and in certain phases of grief and creative work. It is the mode of thought which characterizes the extremes in personal isolation and in personal intimacy.

Although all of these are thought to share the formal properties of primary process, obviously over this range there are differences of meaning and, as yet, largely unformulated differences of thought organization. To some extent there is room for such differences in our understanding that primary process and secondary process are concepts—that no pure forms exist in actuality. In addition, some of the differences are formulated by Kris's concept of regression in the service of the ego (1950), by Rapaport's (1953; 1957b; 1958, p. 739) models of activity and passivity, and by Rapaport's (1951a, pt. 7) and Freud's (1900, chap. 7) concept of a hierarchic layering of thought organization (see also the Freudian passages cited by Rapaport, 1951a, p. 479).

Secondary process refers to the ordinary, ordered, time-space-oriented, logically constrained, language-based, conceptual organization of thought. Although the conceptual organization of thought which characterizes secondary process depends on the internalization of a capacity for active delay, it does not follow that peremptoriness or imperativeness should be a defining characteristic of primary-process function. Although Rapaport (1960a, p. 192) suggested the latter, he also spoke of degrees of peremptoriness (1960a, p. 187). We *can* speak of primitive primary process function as need organized though not necessarily imperative. In the infant, intense need determines an imperative mode. However, there are moments from the first hours of life when the infant is "no longer asleep and not yet in a state of hunger or other distress" (Rapaport,

1960a, p. 230, in reference to observations of Wolff, 1959), when need is not at an imperative level.

Notwithstanding the lack of systematic definitions, which Gill (1967, p. 265) has noted, Freud's concept of primary and secondary process stands as the outstanding generalization of all his early efforts to understand the language of dreams, symptoms, art, jokes, and the psychopathology of everyday life as forms of thought. Since much of the latter part of my paper amounts to variations on the theme of the identity of perception and the identity of thought (Freud, 1900, pp. 566–67, 602), I should emphasize that in contrast to the hallucinatory perceptual identity, the capacity to experience thought identity involves a gradation or differentiation within primary-process functioning—a first step toward realization of the potentiality for secondary-process thought and, at the same time, a first step toward realization of the potentiality for advanced forms of primary-process thought. The capacity established is that of being able to think in images with the realization that those images are not identical with, but represent or refer to, their objects.

The Absent Object

As for the absent object, it is obvious—a point of clear interdisciplinary agreement—that all ideation or thought is the capacity to represent an absent object. Nevertheless, the concept of the absent object and its genealogy—the history of its development from early to advanced forms—occupies a central place in psychoanalytic theory at every level of development. Furthermore, it has a special meaning within psychoanalysis which I believe is crucial to any psychoanalytic contribution to the understanding of language. I shall mention briefly some dimensions of meaning of the absent object.

First of all, it is the absence of the object in the face of need which evokes awareness, and the ideational content of awareness is presumably some fragmentary image of the absent object. A point of interdisciplinary agreement in addition to that mentioned above is that consciousness begins in some form of awareness of the object and not with the inner sources or mechanisms of the mind (Piaget, 1965, p. 47; Freud, 1900, pp. 574, 611, 615–16; Chomsky, 1968, pp. 26, 43, 103, 173). The specific psychoanalytic concept of instinctual drives as the ultimate determinants of behavior (Rapaport, 1960b, pp. 47–49) includes the object as a defining characteristic of instinctual drive (Rapaport, 1960a, p. 202). The idea as representative of a drive is the point where need achieves representation as wish, where memory becomes desire in the form of a recalled fragment of a prior experience of satisfaction with the now absent object.

Internalization of aspects of the relationship with the object structures thought and is the mode of original differentiation from the object, and of subsequent development. Psychoanalysts assume that every subsequent quest, no matter how distantly derivative, is in some way modeled upon the original search for the object.

Of course, originally there *is* no self-conscious search, only a given directionality, and no self and no object as such. For this reason Loewald has recently suggested (1974) that the term *object* should be omitted from discussions of primitive mentation. This could have the advantage of reminding us that there is such a thing as the undifferentiated phase, but it would have the disadvantage of blurring the role of the object—no matter how primitively represented—in what could be called the object organization of both early ideation and advanced thought.

Psychoanalysis and Language

In his essay on interpretation, entitled *Freud and Philosophy*, Paul Ricoeur contends that "the psychoanalyst is a leading participant in any general discussion about language" (1970, p. 4), and that the area of language "is an area today where all philosophical investigations cut across one another" (p. 3). Noam Chomsky has often cited (for example, 1965, p. 8) W. von Humboldt's statement that language can "make infinite use of finite means." Similarly, Ricoeur asks, "How can language be put to such diverse uses as mathematics and myth, physics and art? It is no accident," he continues, "that we ask ourselves this question today. We have at our disposal a symbolic logic, an exegetical science, an anthropology, and a psychoanalysis and, perhaps for the first time, we are able to encompass in a single question the problem of the unification of human discourse" (pp. 3-4).

A number of psychoanalysts have been interested in language, and Edelson (1972) has recently provided us with a study of Freud as a linguist and a detailed comparison of Freud's work with that of Chomsky. Much of Edelson's comparison centers on *The Interpretation of Dreams*. Dreams have a grammar of their own. The dream-work is a form of thinking. Yet the dream, like another language or another symbolic mode, is interpretable because the uniqueness of its own grammar is nevertheless located within a universal grammar, the latter an innate potentiality of every human. We do not, in other words, interpret dreams by use of a dream book which names the meaning of individual images. The possibility of interpretation is not based on the fact that different words in different languages, or different images in different symbolic modes, designate identical entities. Interpretation is based, rather, on as full knowledge as possible of the text of the dream, the primary-process mode of thinking, the patient's past and current reality, and the transference. All of these are essential vantage points from which both analyst and patient take their bearings on the structure and meaning, or the syntax and semantics, of the dream.

Much of the knowledge that allows for the understanding of a dream—the dream-work transformations by which the basic dream thought is pictorially and semantically interpreted—is not and need not be conscious in the mind of either analyst or patient. But when such rules of transformation are said to be known intuitively this does not mean only vaguely or approximately. It is precise but unconscious knowledge of the kind covered by Piaget's (1970) concept of the "cognitive unconscious." It is thus not incumbent upon every psychoanalyst to study linguistics.[1] However, for many of those who do, the structure of language seems to offer the clearest access to an understanding of the structure of mind. Not that the two are identical, but an understanding of language structure promises access to an understanding of the mind in its preverbal and nonverbal, as well as in its verbal, modes of functioning.

This brief indication of the vast scope of the problem of language, hinting at the many possible levels of psychoanalytic contributions toward increased understanding, serves as my general context. I hope now to work my way toward psychoanalytically more familiar ground by way of some comments on the function of abstraction.

Abstraction

Psychoanalysts, committed to a genetic point of view at both phylogenetic and ontogenetic levels, find it difficult to believe that human language is as different from animal thinking as Chomsky maintains, or that it is as similar as Skinner asserts. Chomsky's concept of innatism, we psychoanalysts would say, is limited to the innate ego potentiality for the achievement of language competence, which is revealed in the language performance evoked by contact with a community of speakers. While we would agree that language presupposes innate ego factors specific to humans, psychoanalytic innatism would add the assumption of the phylogenetically older instinctual drives,

---

1. One is reminded here of Waelder's (1962, p. 620) assertion at a different level that perfectly competent clinical psychoanalytic work can be carried out by an analyst who has no particular conscious grasp of the most general level of psychoanalytic theory.

which interact with ego, superego, and external reality in the phylogenetic shaping and the ontogenetic evoking of the specifically human linguistic function. The difference is the emphasis on instinctual drive and superego factors, both of which are intimately associated with the absent or renounced object. The cardinal similarity between Chomsky and psychoanalytic thought is in regarding language—and ego function generally—as a system of competence.

Saussure, like all linguists since, warned against the common tendency to regard language as a "naming process only—a list of words, each corresponding to the thing that it names" (1966, p. 65). The two elements, the idea and the sound image, in what Saussure called the linguistic sign, are both psychological. The idea is the concept or abstraction and would correspond to Freud's thing-representation. The sound image is the word-representation. The two form a unity, each evoking the other. Saussure called the sound (or graphic or other sensuous image) the signifier and the concept the signified. So we can have in mind a triangle. The apex would be the signified, meaning the concept or the abstraction; the lower left-hand corner the signifier, meaning the sound or other sensuous image; the lower right-hand corner the referent or object, meaning the event or entity to which the concept refers.

This triangle—and particularly the apex of the triangle, the point of abstraction—models a basic characteristic of language and provides a means of considering the differences in human and animal thinking. For Chomsky, the differences are phylogenetic givens in the form of a uniquely human potentiality for language competence. Although not guilty of Piaget's (1971, pp. 89–90) accusation of all-or-none innatism—he repeatedly acknowledges the necessity of experiential releasing factors[2]—Chomsky does seem impatient with attempts to trace

2. In the reference cited, Piaget wrote that Chomsky "sees only two alternatives—either an innate schema that governs with necessity, or acquisition from outside."

precursors of human speech in animals. Perhaps from having long contended with Skinner's pigeons, he is also apt to write off reported conversations with dolphins as science fiction. In sum, and for good reason, he does not have great faith that a genetic hypothesis or a genetic study can avoid the genetic fallacy.

In general, however, there is agreement that one factor which distinguishes human from animal thinking is the degree and/or kind of abstraction, a faculty probably related to the relative lack of pre-set instinctual patterning and the long dependency period in humans. The lack of pre-set instinctual patterning may be considered a kind of "leeway" specific to humans. The leeway should not be understood as a realm of sheer chaos. It implies, instead, a different set of innate potentialities involving a longer dependency period and a more crucial role for the object in the gradual formation of the human capacity for abstraction. That which humans and animals share is the use of indices and signals. Presumably, at this level of functioning the apex of the triangle—abstraction or concept formation—is lost and the signifier as index or signal directly signifies the referent. Edelson (1972), in accord with Piaget, defines index as a signifier "intrinsically attached to what it signifies (e.g., the 'footprint' that signifies or indicates 'elephant is proximate')," and signal as a signifier "arbitrarily attached to what it automatically—that is, without mediation by abstraction—signifies (e.g., the 'bell' that in

---

However, the "invariant properties of human language" (Chomsky, 1971, p. 23) which, according to Chomsky's hypothesis, reflect innate properties of mind, still require experience to be brought into operation (pp. 15, 18, 21, 23, 43). It may be said that Piaget does question more specifically than Chomsky the meaning of innateness. His point is that "even when a trait is recognized as hereditary, the question of its formation remains." He emphasizes equilibration processes that yield necessities in accordance with "the general laws of organization by which the self-regulation of behavior is governed" (p. 90) and adds that "the acquisition of language presupposes the prior formation of sensori-motor intelligence, which goes to justify Chomsky's ideas concerning the necessity of a prelinguistic substrate akin to rationality" (p. 91).

conditioning signifies or signals 'dinner is proximate')" (p. 274).

I say that "presumably" the apex of the triangle is lost at this level of functioning because that does seem the consensus. However, it is difficult for me to think of any mental activity utterly devoid of abstraction. I would prefer to think of a hierarchy of levels, or perhaps simply different degrees and kinds of abstraction. In part, this distinction has already been made (see Edelson, p. 273), in that abstractions may be either configurative (imaged) or conceptual. Langer (1942) writes of the primitive conception as contrasted with the definitive concept of discursive language; Piaget (1945), of preconceptual representation and concepts. But I would suggest some kind of abstractive step is involved even at the level of signals and indices, which Langer, although using a slightly different terminology, calls "the very first manifestations of mind" (1942, p. 22)—some notion, that is, if not of an object of danger or gratification, then of danger or gratification as such, no matter how primitively conceived, and no doubt not consciously experienced.

But what is abstraction and what characterizes the uniquely human abstractive function? Although Edelson would like to limit the term *representative* to the signifier, leaving the concept as that which is signified, in the psychoanalytic tradition the idea or concept is also a level of representation.[3] Conceptual representation is abstraction. To illustrate degrees or levels of conceptualization or abstraction, let me begin with a statement of Langer's on signals and signs.

> Man, unlike all other animals, uses "signs" not only to *indicate* things, but also to *represent* them. To a clever dog,

---

3. Rapaport (1957a, 2:270) and Loewald (1971, p. 107) recognize two levels of representation. Instinct as such is the "psychical representative" of organic stimuli. Instinct, in turn, can be represented as the idea—a "drive representation." Actually, both conceive of multiple levels of representation. Loewald wrote, "Mental or psychical representatives are hierarchically structured in such a way that representatives of a lower order can be rerepresented . . . on higher mental levels."

the name of a person is a signal that the person is present; you say the name, he pricks up his ears and looks for its object. If you say "dinner," he becomes restive, expecting food. You cannot make any communication to him that is not taken as a signal of something immediately forthcoming. His mind is a simple and direct *transmitter* of messages from the world to his motor centers. With man it is different. We use certain "signs" among ourselves that do not point to anything in our actual surroundings. Most of our words are not signs in the sense of signals. They are used to talk *about* things, not to direct our eyes and ears and noses toward them. Instead of announcers of things, they are reminders. They have been called "substitute signs," for in our present experience they take the place of things that we have perceived in the past, or even things that we can merely imagine by combining memories, things that *might* be in past or future experience . . . such "signs" . . . serve . . . to let us develop a characteristic attitude toward objects *in absentia,* which is called "thinking of" or "referring to" what is not here. [1942, p. 24]

Here the degree of abstraction is a function of the distance or autonomy of the concept from its referent, dependent on the progression from primitive to advanced modes of thought organization (Rapaport, 1951b, pp. 422–23).

In primitive mentation, the memorial fragment of a prior experience of satisfaction evoked by recurrence of need and presumably experienced as though it is an actual repetition of the experience—the identity of perception—is a protoconception. In relation to this level, the ideational component of the identity of thought, a conception, is a further abstractive step involving the realization that the image of the object and the object it refers to are separate. Further abstractive and organizing steps occur as responses in a system in which drives and objects are being mutually constituted (Loewald, 1971, pp. 117–20); objects are automatically categorized as objects of need, objects of danger, or relatively neutral. Such primitive automatic categorization is prior to, and indeed the presupposition of, grammatical categories and the higher-level categorization of objects.

Primitive Mentation and the Psychoanalytic Theory of Language Acquisition

I shall now review a few additional dimensions of primitive mentation as these pertain to language and to some of Peter Wolff's (1967) observations on a psychoanalytic theory of language acquisition.

An image—I use the word broadly as relating to any sense datum, not just the visual—is first of all a percept. A remembered percept is an idea—that is, an image evoked by a situation which does not include every aspect of the stimulus situation that originally evoked the percept. Primitive imperative ideation, presumably in the form of images identical with random and partial perceptual aspects of the experience of prior satisfaction, is evoked by a situation of intense need. At such a primitive level, the ideation that represents the present need also represents the object and is simultaneously both memory and prototypical anticipation (of the object of satisfaction). The sequence portrays elements of the situation which preordain subsequent development of conceptual I-object differentiation within past, present, and future temporal dimensions.

Psychoanalytic genetic epistemology accents the situation of basic need and the way in which all of development is anaclitic in relation to it. Consciousness begins with perceptual (and affective) responses. However, the memories of such percepts are not randomly recorded but are organized in terms of the action patterns which coordinate need and object.

Although in many ways compatible with this, the work of

Piaget derives from development as observed in nonimperative situations. He consequently pays more attention to the external sources of disequilibrium together with their cognitive-structural resolution, and less attention to inner sources of disequilibrium, to what he has (unfortunately) termed "the affective unconscious" (Piaget, 1970), and to affect as such.

The psychoanalytic model suggests that primitive imperative ideation is of hallucinatory vividness; and there is at least *some* reason to assume that it is, on the basis of direct observation of infants (Holt, 1967), inference from dreams, and certain pathological conditions understood as regressive. There are several points to be made about this suggestion. First of all, whether or not imperative ideation is of hallucinatory vividness is not essential to the model. Secondly, the model is not tied to a point in time when the infant (or foetus) is first capable of ideation. Thirdly, if ideation of hallucinatory vividness does occur in the first year of life, it is likely that it results from both the intensity of the need and the infant's lack of the kind of developed control or differentiation that would allow representation to stop short of hallucination—namely, at the memory. An early phase of minimal need may evoke imagery of less than hallucinatory vividness—perhaps of varying degrees of vividness, depending at first on the intensity of need and later on both the intensity of need and developed controls.

Wolff (1967) and Holt (1967), basing their ideas on the work of Piaget, largely (but see Wolff, p. 326) reject the possibility of early infantile hallucination because of the "essentially veridical memory traces implied" (Holt, p. 371). It seems to me that both Wolff and Holt do unwarranted violence to Rapaport's teaching in this regard by ignoring what Rapaport (and Freud) assumed to be the nature of primitive ideation. Wolff's suggestion that the idea of an "isomorphism between the physical event and the child's experience of it" (1967, p. 308) is "the position of classic psychoanalytic theory" is simply not true.

"Does the child," Wolff asks, "perceive the tension-reducing event as a breast-object that affords pleasure, or the act of sucking as a spatio-temporally fixed interaction between his mouth and an external object?" The answer of classic psychoanalytic theory would be, in a word, no, notwithstanding the fact that locutions close to this often characterize the average analyst's shorthand way of employing the primary model. To elaborate—and here I only paraphrase a passage from Rapaport, a passage that Wolff incorrectly cites (p. 308) as though it were a correction rather than an explication of Freud's thought—it depends on what is meant by "object." If what is meant is representation of the object already constituted as object and other, it is too much to ask of an infant, awake or asleep. Primitive hallucination, if it occurs, as well as ideation short of hallucinatory vividness, must be understood as much less organized than this; it is more like a fused fragment of the prior perceptual experience, such as sensation in the lips or warmth of cheek, an odor, a ray of light, a wisp of hair, a creaking door, or the sound of a voice. Or it might be even less cognitive than the memory of any such fused fragment—an experience of recollection so diffuse as to be the memory of an affect, the latter a case where the lines between memory, hallucination, and affective response become murky indeed.

Although Wolff and Holt presumably base their reasoning about early ideation on the work of Piaget, it has not been shown that Piaget's basic assumptions about early mentation are incompatible with ideation representing an absent object of need. True enough, such objects would not be conceived "as entities in themselves, but only as functional elements (things . . . merely as something to be sucked, something to be swung or handled, etc.)" (Piaget, 1937, p. 162). It may be assumed

that the objects imaged in absence are those correlative with
needs or internally initiated disequilibrium (for example,
"something to be sucked"). It is less likely that "unsought"
external objects which themselves initiate disequilibrium in
the form of interest (for example, "something to be swung")
would be imaged. In any event, primitive representation of
whatever functional elements would be of the fragmentary
nature described above. Of course, there would be no "perma-
nent objects" and no "objective organization of space" (p.
160), but the structuralization necessary for such concepts
presupposes some kind of prior ideation pertaining to an
absent object of need, no matter how primitively represented.[4]

Wolff acknowledges "that the developmental principles of
psychoanalysis contradict any pure association or conditioning
psychology because they postulate inherent forces (drives) and
structures (defenses) which codetermine the apperception of
the external world" (p. 312). However, in asserting "how
intimately in classic psychoanalytic theory the associationist
concept of memory was linked to a formulation of language
acquisition" (p. 312), he cites those passages where Freud
(1895, pp. 421–22; 1915, pp. 201–02; 1923, p. 20), according
to Rapaport (1957a, p. 159), "went hog-wild" in giving verbal
traces a paramount role in preconscious function, and does not
cite the passage where Freud (1940 [1938], pp. 161–64)
withdrew this formulation.

Of course we are all aware, at times, of nameless percepts,
affects, and unformed, preverbal concepts, so it cannot be

4. Edelson (1972) is a bit more careful in his phrasing. Explicitly, he sees dreaming
as dependent on language competence. However, when he asserts that "a principal
implication of Freud's use of the rebus as a model of the dream is that the latent
dream thoughts must be, to begin with, represented linguistically or must come to be
represented linguistically before a manifest dream can be constructed" (pp. 270–71),
he implicitly makes dreaming dependent on language performance, a wholly
untenable position. Even language competence as an innate species-specific capacity
would still undergo formation over time and involve primitive phases.

argued that we can only be conscious of that which we have a word for, as though all that is involved is the simple naming. To be fully conscious of something is to be aware of an event or entity and of its relationship with other events and entities in our world (Rapaport, 1957b, p. 422, and repeatedly elsewhere). Consciousness at anything beyond a primitive perceptual level requires an organization of experience. Language is the paramount means and reflection of the human capacity for such organization. I believe this is what Freud was attempting to express at the time when the preconscious was conceived as a system, in his references to the relationship between consciousness and the word-representation.

Now, to summarize the relevance of this discussion on primitive mentation to my topic, the ego differentiates from external reality and from the id by means of preverbal thought and action. A wish names an object, an external reality, and also a need, an internal reality. At the same time, even at a primary-process level, it names a relationship between need and object. The action pattern which fulfills the need confirms the differentiation of need, action, and object, and a first orientation is established. I would suggest that the sequence of this adaptive system has the structure of a sentence, and even though still at a level shared with animals, it might well codetermine, with other factors, basic components of human grammar. The need is the "I" or noun phrase, and the action and object the verb phrase anlage. Of course, it is the object which is primitively imaged. The action is automatic and the I, as such, is silent; in other words, the need is only represented by virtue of imaging the object. This would accord with de Laguna's (1927, cited by McNeill, 1970, p. 1076) suggestion that the one-word, holophrastic speech of early childhood is predicative, and also with the Freud, Chomsky, and Piaget references cited in the earlier discussion of the absent object, regarding the peripheral focus of early consciousness.

Nonimperative Mentation, Play, and the Meaning
of the Arbitrariness of the Signifier

In turning to the specifically human capacity for higher-level abstraction, I would like to consider a different phase of primitive mentation. Freud's model of mind (1900, chap. 7), elaborated by Rapaport (1951a, pp. 689–730) in terms of the primary models of thought, affect, and action, reflects and fosters a tendency toward exclusive emphasis on the peremptory or imperative aspects of early behavior; such behavior is later delayed and eventually tamed through a variety of responses to the absence of the object. The model might be thought to ignore early nonimperative behavior,[5] a kind of behavior that I believe is particularly important as a formative basis in the appearance of language. In his 1905 "Jokes and their Relation to the Unconscious," nonimperative primary-process functioning was described by Freud as follows:

> If we do not require our mental apparatus at the moment for supplying one of our indispensable satisfactions, we allow it itself to work in the direction of pleasure from its own activity. I suspect that this is in general the condition that governs all aesthetic ideation. [pp. 95–96]

This brings me to the topic of play, which I would like to associate with the arbitrariness of the signifier in language.

The symbol—the signifier of what Langer (1942, p. 79) calls "presentational symbolism"—has some intrinsic connection with the concept or conception it represents. The sign—the signifier of the language of conceptual or discursive thought—is wholly arbitrary in function, regardless of its origin. This is witnessed not merely by the fact that different words in different languages can represent the same concept, but also by the fact that in each language the relationship of word and

5. The model might also be thought to ignore advanced, active, ego-dominant imperative behavior, a topic which I cannot here pursue.

concept is by arbitrary assignment, without which language as a system and individual language acquisition would not be possible.

The very word *arbitrary* is apt to evoke skepticism among psychoanalysts. "The arbitrary," as Freud put it, "has no existence in mental life" (1909, p. 102). Freud was there rejecting the idea of anything outside the realm of determinism. But the arbitrary, in the sense of a rule of convention, is not undetermined. Were it possible to have full access to the developmental history of any language, then we would know what determined the choice of its every word. We *can* know something about the determinants of a few words, for instance, as illustrated in Roman Jakobson's (1968) account of "Why 'Mama' and 'Papa'?". Or, to cite another example, perhaps both the gesture and word *yes* and the gesture and word *no* derive from the fact that muscular movements of the former are compatible with the acceptance, and of the latter with the rejection, of food. Or, to be utterly fanciful, perhaps there was a primitive arboreal beast which made the sound "Arr" in such a fashion as to have determined the words "arbor" and, eventually, "arboreal." If it were possible to confirm such speculations, they would constitute interesting bits of historical information but in no way account for language as a system. Questions of determinacy of the kind just mentioned recede into insignificance; the issue is that of the determining factors in the human capacity to assign or accept an arbitrary relation between word and concept regardless of the particular elements—some of them completely trivial—which entered into the derivation of the word.

"The slight nasal murmur, the only phonation which can be produced when the lips are pressed to mother's breast or the feeding bottle and the mouth is full," may be, as Jakobson (1968, p. 542) suggests, the phonetic precursor of "mama" or the *m*-form designating "mother" in many languages. But, for approximately a year in the evolution of this *m*-interjection it does not yet designate mother. It occurs "as an anticipatory signal at the mere sight of food and finally as a manifestation of a desire to eat, or more generally, as an expression of discontent and impatient longing for missing food or absent nurser or any ungranted wish" (p. 542).

At the point where *mama* can actually designate mother—the transition point for the word from what Jakobson calls "affective expression to designative language" (p. 543)—a clear concept of mother has been formed. We speak of psychological differentiation of the mother-child unit and of established object constancy. Clear concept formation—clear differentiation of concept and referent—also implies a realization at some level of a clear differentiation of concept and signifier—namely, that any particular signifier is not innately necessary to, or a part of, the concept. To realize, even though not consciously, that a concept could as well be represented by another signifier, is to realize the arbitrariness of the assignment regardless of the determinants in the origin of the signifier in a particular language. It is, at the same time, the abstractive step that allows for the active invention in play and fantasy of arbitrary signifiers; the invention of concepts; and, to a limited extent, even the invention of idiosyncratic grammars. It is the step which ushers in the period of seemingly effortless multilanguage learning.

Langer emphasized the human tendency to babble—to play with sounds—as a precursor of language. Playing with sounds is, psychologically speaking, to play with sound images. I suggest that similarly, at a slightly later phase, children also play with conceptions and concepts. Although clear concept formation (which implies me/not me and a host of simultaneous inter- and intrastructural differentiations) allows for a higher-level conceptual play, it may be that the prior tendency to play, reflecting the instinctual leeway and the cared-for situation, also is a factor in the formation of clear concepts and the discovery of the arbitrary, conventional nature of the signifier. If so, the leeway that allows for play, the capacity to take a distance and occupy various conceptual vantage points in relation to objects of interest, would not only be a condition governing "all aesthetic ideation," as Freud (1905, p. 96) wrote, it would also be a formative presupposition of the capacity for conceptual thought.[6]

The Complementarity of Imperative and Nonimperative Modes in the Organization of Thought

The anlage of play in primitive mentation would occur in phases of minor psychological disequilibrium—where the pressure of "indispensable needs" is, in Rapaport's terms (1960a, p. 187), at a low degree of peremptoriness. Dreaming, as well as being a mode of thought, could be considered a mode of play. But what I have in mind here is the likelihood of a freer kind of perception and ideation in the brief periods of wakefulness before and after feeding—before needs have mounted to imperative level and following their fulfillment.

We assume that at a moment of intense need the infant is initially compelled to focus on percepts at hand and subsequently on images representing prior experiences of satisfaction. But the imperative act of attending under pressure of need, though intense, would for that very reason have less opportunity for awareness of conceptual relationships. The intensity of focus would allow no leeway for comparing the object of perception or ideation with prior experience or what had been anticipated. Changing features of perception or

6. If this interpretation of arbitrariness is correct, Jakobson's work has not thrown doubt on the "complete arbitrariness of the verbal sign," as Piaget (1971, p. 78) suggests. Furthermore, Saussure's distinction of the "relatively" and the "radically arbitrary," which Piaget mentions in the same passage, would not hold. Organization and arbitrariness are not at opposite poles. The systematic character of language does not limit arbitrariness, as Saussure wrote (1966, p. 79). On the contrary, arbitrariness of the verbal sign is an essential aspect of language as a system. To use Saussure's example, *dix-neuf* may have a more obvious history of origin, but in its function of signifying a certain number, it is as radically arbitrary as *dix* or *neuf*.

ideation would not be understood or integrated as various aspects of the same object. Each feature, under the pressure of need, would be the straw grasped at the moment to the exclusion of all else. Presumably, it is the nonimperative situation which allows for the possibility of noticing various aspects of what is at present perceived, and of making primitive comparisons, at the same time, with the recalled and the anticipated. Although we assume that basic needs ultimately compel the organization of thought, the accomplishment of that organization largely occurs when the pressure of need is minimal, when affective response can function at a signal level, and when the scope of consciousness permits a field of perception or a train of ideas to be experienced.

I here contrast the imperative and nonimperative modes only to suggest their complementarity in the organization of thought and the ultimate dependency of both on the actual, the recalled, or the anticipated absence of the object. The precursor of trust implied in primitive nonimperative modes would have no such meaning except in the context of the recalled or anticipated absence of the object.

The Conceptual and Symbolic Modes

The ordinary contrast between symbolic (presentational) and conceptual (discursive) modes of thought does not coincide with the contrast between imperative and nonimperative. Symbolic and conceptual thought can each occur in either the imperative or the nonimperative mode.

In primitive mentation symbolic and conceptual thought are not yet differentiated. In advanced thinking the differentiation is not, first of all, in the signifiers but in the nature of their objects and in the motive and style of abstraction—that is, the signified—evoked by the nature of the object. Although both are ultimately evoked by absence of the object, both are also sustained by the actual, recalled, or anticipated presence of the object. Deprivation in the absence of the object can be known as such only by recall or anticipation of gratification and presence of the object; gratification, only by recall or anticipation of deprivation and absence of the object. The locus in primitive thinking of the absent object becomes in advanced thinking—whether symbolic or conceptual—that of any compelling or interesting unknown or unattained. The characterizing method of the conceptual mode is to organize and build on that which is consciously known; that of the symbolic, to represent that which is consciously unknown. The formal properties of secondary process predominate in the former and those of primary process in the latter.

To conceptualize primary-process functioning as a style of relatively direct response to the unknown, conforms with the dominance of primary process in primitive functioning and the tendency toward it in regressive functioning and in dreaming, without assuming the converse—namely, that all primary-process functioning is primitive or regressive.

Freud (1900, p. 602) wrote:

> There is yet another reason for which . . . the second system is obliged to correct the primary process. . . . Thinking must concern itself with the connecting paths between ideas, without being led astray by the *intensities* of those ideas. But it is obvious that condensations of ideas, as well as intermediate and compromise structures, must obstruct the attainment of the identity aimed at. Since they substitute one idea for another, they cause a deviation from the path which would have led on from the first idea. Processes of this kind are therefore scrupulously avoided in secondary thinking. It is easy to see, too, that the unpleasure principle, which in other respects supplies the thought-process with its most important signposts, puts difficulties in its path towards establishing "thought identity." Accordingly, thinking must aim at

freeing itself more and more from exclusive regulation by the unpleasure principle and at restricting the development of affect in thought-activity to the minimum required for acting as a signal.

I see this as meaning that to the extent a project calls for secondary-process thought, primary process is a breakdown, possibly a regressive avoidance, and at least temporarily an interference. The issue not addressed in the passage cited is that to the extent a project calls for primary-process thought, secondary process is avoidance, the latter a classic obsessional defense: in Eliot's (1919, p. 10) aphorism, "The bad poet is usually unconscious where he ought to be conscious, and conscious where he ought to be unconscious."

Summary

I have throughout the above discussion attempted to thematize the role of the absent object in the evocation of language and thought, and to specify in that context some of the experiential factors crucial to realization of the innate human potentiality for language. My intention has largely been to relate Freud's primary model of mind to certain nonimperative aspects of experience more adequately accounted for in the thought of Piaget and current linguistics. In addition, I have underlined the known relevance of the Freudian model to imperative aspects of experience not accounted for by Piaget or linguistics, and have indicated the interdependence of the imperative and nonimperative in the establishment of the conceptual organization of thought. Finally, I have suggested that primary-process functioning does not necessarily imply regression, and that symbolization —a mode in which the signifier represents both a known and unknown signified—is a possible response to the unknown at every hierarchic level.

168   LANGUAGE AND THE GENEALOGY OF THE ABSENT OBJECT

REFERENCES

Chomsky, N. *Aspects of the Theory of Syntax.* Cambridge: M.I.T. Press, 1965.
————. *Language and Mind.* New York: Harcourt Brace Jovanovich, 1968.
————. *Problems of Knowledge and Freedom.* New York: Pantheon Books (Random House), 1971.
Edelson, M. "Language and Dreams." *Psychoanalytic Study of the Child* 27 (1972): 203–82.
Eliot, T. S. "Tradition and the Individual Talent" (1919). In *Selected Essays.* New York: Harcourt Brace, 1950.
Freud, S. "Project for a Scientific Psychology" (1895). In *The Origins of Psycho-Analysis: Letters to Wilhelm Fliess, Drafts and Notes, 1887–1902.* New York: Basic Books, 1954.
————. *Standard Edition of the Complete Psychological Works.* London: Hogarth, 1953–64:
  The Interpretation of Dreams (1900), vol. 5.
  Jokes and their Relation to the Unconscious (1905), vol. 8.
  "Analysis of a Phobia in a Five-Year-Old Boy" (1909), vol. 10.
  "The Unconscious" (1915), vol. 14.
  Beyond the Pleasure Principle (1920), vol. 18.
  The Ego and the Id (1923), vol. 19.
  An Outline of Psycho-analysis (1940 [1938]), vol. 23.
Gill, M. "The Primary Process." *Psychological Issues* 5 (1967): 260–98.
Holt, R. "The Development of the Primary Process: A Structural View." *Psychological Issues* 5 (1967):345–83.
Jakobson, R. "Why, 'Mama' and 'Papa'?" *Selected Writings*, vol. 1. The Hague: Mouton, 1968.
Kris, E. "On Preconscious Mental Processes." *Psychoanalytic Quarterly* 19 (1950): 540–60.
de Laguna, G. A. *Speech: Its Function and Development.* Bloomington, Ind.: Indiana University Press, 1927.
Langer, S. *Philosophy in a New Key* (1942). New York: New American Library, Mentor paperback, 1948.
Loewald, H. "On Motivation and Instinct Theory." *Psychoanalytic Study of the Child* 26 (1971): 91–128.

———. "Perspectives on Memory." Address delivered to Washington Psychoanalytic Society, Sept. 13, 1974.

McNeill, D. "The Development of Language." In *Leonard Carmichael's Manual of Child Psychology*, 3d ed. Edited by P. H. Mussen. New York: Wiley, 1970.

Piaget, J. "Principal Factors Determining Intellectual Evolution from Childhood to Adult Life" (1937), trans. and commentary by D. Rapaport. In D. Rapaport, *Organization and Pathology of Thought.* New York: Columbia University Press, 1951.

———. *Play, Dreams and Imitation in Childhood* (1945). New York: Norton, 1962.

———. *Insights and Illusions of Philosophy* (1965). Translated by W. Mays. New York: World Publishing Company, 1971.

———. "The Affective Unconscious and the Cognitive Unconscious." Address at fall meeting, American Psychoanalytic Association, 1970. Published version, *Journal of the American Psychoanalytic Association* 21 (1973): 249–61.

———. *Structuralism.* New York: Harper Torchbooks, 1971.

Rapaport, D. *Organization and Pathology of Thought.* New York: Columbia University Press, 1951a.

———. "The Conceptual Model of Psychoanalysis" (1951b). In *The Collected Papers of David Rapaport*, ed. M. M. Gill. New York: Basic Books, 1967.

———. "Some Metapsychological Considerations Concerning Activity and Passivity" (1953). In *The Collected Papers of David Rapaport*, ed. M. M. Gill. New York: Basic Books, 1967.

———. *Seminars on Elementary Metapsychology.* Seminars at Austen Riggs Center, ed. S. C. Miller. Mimeographed, 1957a.

———. "The Theory of Ego Autonomy: A Generalization" (1957b). In *The Collected Papers of David Rapaport*, ed. M. M. Gill. New York: Basic Books, 1967.

———. "A Historical Survey of Psychoanalytic Ego Psychology" (1958). In *The Collected Papers of David Rapaport*, ed. M. M. Gill. New York: Basic Books, 1967.

———. "On the Psychoanalytic Theory of Motivation." In *Nebraska Symposium on Motivation*, vol. 8, ed. M. Jones. University of Nebraska Press, 1960a.

Rapaport, D. *The Structure of Psychoanalytic Theory, Psychological Issues* 2, no. 2, Monograph 6, 1960b.

Ricoeur, P. *Freud and Philosophy*. Translated by D. Savage. New Haven: Yale University Press, 1970.

de Saussure, F. *Course in General Linguistics*. Edited by C. Bally and A. Riedlinger, translated by W. Baskin. New York; McGraw-Hill, 1966.

Waelder, R. "Psychoanalysis, Scientific Method, and Philosophy." *Journal of the American Psychoanalytic Assn.* 10 (1962): 617–37.

Wolff, P. "Observations on Newborn Infants," *Psychosomatic Medicine* 21 (1959): 110–18.

———. "Cognitive Considerations for a Psychoanalytic Theory of Language Acquisition." *Psychological Issues* 5 (1967): 300–43.

Psychiatry and Human Affairs

8

The Family, Myth, and Ethics

THEODORE LIDZ

During these times that try men's souls—when our democracy is threatened with destruction by the corruption of power and wealth that poisons the body politic—I, like many others, have been preoccupied with the perversion of ethical principles by our leaders and the consequent alienation of our youth, as well as with the weakened national ethos, which leaves us without collective purpose and direction.

While attention and concern have been directed to the transformations of the world brought about by the scientific and industrial revolutions, and more specifically to the hopes and fears raised by the atomic and computer revolutions, a reorientation of man's understanding of himself has been emerging that may affect man's ways of life even more profoundly than other aspects of the scientific revolution. Like all such profound reorientations, it disrupts established institutions and mores and raises threats of chaos; and to many it may seem catastrophic rather than progressive. It relates to the awareness that ethnic differences are primarily cultural rather than racial. It arises from the belief not only that all men are created more or less equal but also that what a person becomes depends very largely on how and where he is brought up. It derives from the conviction that a child requires a developmental milieu that provides certain essential nurture, structuring, and socialization to enable him to become a useful and reasonably secure adult.

173

Such concepts first took root in the United States, where it became obvious that children reared in the new setting could differ profoundly from their immigrant parents, and blossomed as changes occurred in underprivileged peoples throughout the world. The ductility of the infant was seen to be far greater than could be imagined in relatively static societies with set social hierarchies. The reorientation, however, has come about primarily through man's expansion of his scientific scrutiny of nature to include himself, and his subsequent efforts to change and improve himself by scientific rather than religious means.

The belief in the malleability of man relates, of course, to the Jeffersonian emphasis on education, to the Marxist belief in the effects of economic oppression, to Jesuit and Communist faith in early indoctrination, to Pavlovian studies of the effects of conditioning; and it depends upon the Freudian recognition of the importance of the emotional atmosphere of the early developmental setting and of the internalization of parental models. Yet it is more than any of these or all of these. It concerns the importance of the total developmental setting, cultural as well as economic, cognitive as well as emotional, and intrafamilial as well as societal, for both the new recruits born into the society and the future of the society (Lidz, 1972).

The new belief in the potential of all men if reared properly in a culturally rich environment opens the way for a truer democracy than any envisioned by the founding fathers of our country or by those who led the French and Communist revolutions. Although still far from realization, the belief has enabled disadvantaged ethnic groups to find hope and gain self-esteem that may be the essential precursors of achievement. The new vision has engendered discontent and upheavals throughout the world. It challenges caste systems, implicit as well as explicit, which have been major guides to what niches in society children are reared to fill. It challenges basic assumptions about the individual's responsibility for finding opportunity for himself and for providing a proper setting in which to raise his children.

Such tasks cannot devolve upon the individual or the family alone; for only the larger society can assure many children of an adequate social and economic setting. The ideal of equal opportunity, though superb, may be beyond realization even if the vast social reforms it would require are enacted. Carried to a logical conclusion, the ideal implies that no child should have any environmental advantage over another, including the educational and emotional attributes of parents. Even if all families were made equal economically, they could not be made to offer equal emotional, cognitive, and cultural opportunities. Yet it seems highly improbable that any setting that does not rely upon the family can be suitable for raising children.

A profound challenge to traditional ethical standards accompanies the emphasis on the importance of the early physical and emotional environment in shaping the personality. Poverty is not the fault of the individual but reflects the way in which the established society plays favorites. Criminality is not a moral problem and reason for disgrace or punishment, but the consequence of socioeconomic or emotional deprivation in childhood. Should heroin addiction be punished or treated? Why does society blame and punish its victims? Samuel Butler (1872) raised this issue a hundred years ago: the criminals in his mythical *Erewhon* were treated by Straighteners (perhaps the first conceptualization of a psychotherapist), whereas those ill with tuberculosis were severely punished for endangering others. Currently, some black activists are teaching that black hold-up men and even black murderers are political prisoners rather than criminals, because the "establishment's" discrimination against their race is responsible for the disadvantaged childhoods and embittered attitudes toward society that lie at the roots of the crimes.

Recognition of the relativity of cultural standards and values has also led to a distrust of established ways and a turning away from them. Not only are we often controlled by the machines we create, but we also ponder whether the societal system, or man who created it, is in control. Eichmann claimed he was not guilty of genocide but simply acted as a loyal citizen of his country. According to a large proportion of American citizens, the soldiers who carried out the massacre at My Lai were only following orders as soldiers. Nor are we to blame for Hiroshima and Nagasaki—we were only preventing the deaths of our own soldiers. However, these very deeds have helped to create the persons we have become and the disillusionment of the subsequent generation that has undermined our national ethos.

And thus, people, particularly the young, not only grasp the relativity of cultural ways but tend to challenge all traditional ways and traditional values. The family is seen as the source of most—if not all—social evils and the belief emerges that it should be replaced by new institutions. The intense attachment of a mother to her child, which has smothered so many children, should be diluted, if not replaced, by a sharing of the maternal role among various females—and males—in a commune. More marriages are unhappy than happy, and therefore the worth of any legal union between couples is challenged, and then discarded by some. As sexual repression causes neuroses, some parents encourage their children to start having sexual relationships at puberty. As adolescents are better educated than their parents, parents doubt their right to foist their values upon their offspring. Such challenges to established ways are congruent with the rebellious tendencies of youth seeking liberation from ties to parents; they echo loudly, and are not refuted readily without resort to dogma and passion. We hear that ethical principles are relative, just part of a mythology, superstition, and prejudice that limit self-expression and prevent the fulfillment of innate potentialities.

Because the scientific use of intellect has brought us to the present impasse, some find science and technology at fault and wish to turn from science, to fall back on faith, to trust in impulses, and to embrace unregenerate nature and become part of it rather than seek to mold it to our purposes and upset its balance. It is enticing to believe that civilization—including the repression it requires—is the source of our woes (Freud, 1930) and that unfettered children would flower to realize innate potentialities. But babies do not become persons without nurturance, structuring, socialization, and enculturation. Too few realize that all societies develop and sustain certain basic taboos, customs, and institutions because they are vital to human stability and security and to the maintenance of a social system without which man is only an animal with limited range and resources.

Although much of the dismay expressed over where "science" has led us tends to disregard how much we have gained from scientific methodology, we may usefully examine whether there have not been shortcomings in our scientific thinking. There is reason to heed complaints that science has brought knowledge but not wisdom, and to ponder the renewal of interest in the mystical and the mythic. Even though the mystical is thought to concern the supernatural, I believe that, in essence, it seeks intuitive knowledge and that which derives from preconscious and unconscious mental processes rather than the reasoned ones. Before we conclude that mores based upon the mythic rest upon superstition, we may do well to consider if mythic thinking might not contribute to the expansion of our scientific thought by making it more pertinent to the study of human affairs and human nature.

Myths fulfill many functions. They seek to account for the ritual that man has used in his efforts to keep nature on its course, and to explain the regularities and inconsistencies of nature; they relate man to his supernatural forebears, creating and preserving genealogies; they magnify the great deeds of ancestors to furnish a people with a sense of distinction and distinctness; and they perform other, related functions for a people by explaining the origins of their universe and themselves. One of the most significant functions of mythology, however, concerns the controlling of acts that would threaten the foundations of society—a function that would seem to derive from efforts to control the vicissitudes of nature.

Ritual was once man's primary way of attempting to keep nature in order. He sought to influence nature by sympathetic magic: ritual copulation in the fields with the May Queen or the Earth Priestess would assure the fertility of the soil; the Yule fires he lit would cause the days to lengthen before the dragon of darkness of the northern winter could completely engulf the earth. Man lived in awe of nature and learned to subject himself to its rule of immutable recurrences; but nature was also dangerously fickle, and he sought to control its fickleness by various rituals, which even included the sacrifice of the king, his son, or some other substitute for him.

Prescientific man—and even more, preliterate man—much like the young child today, understood nature in animistic terms. Piaget's insights into the thinking of the child (Piaget, 1929) provide helpful analogies: the young child thinks "preoperationally" and considers that inanimate objects have wills, motives, and the power to carry out their wishes. The sun rises because it is tired of sleeping; the trees sway in order to fan the clouds to move, and so forth. The child believes that objects in nature were created by men and for men; that wishes can control nature; that his parents can influence natural phenomena, etc. Preliterate man similarly anthropomorphized nature—that is, he understood acts of nature in the only way he could, in terms of human motivations. Anthropomorphization permitted him to do something about controlling natural phenomena. Anthropomorphized nature could be conceived of as gods, giants, or demons who could be influenced by magic, prayer, or sacrifice, or could be appeased or threatened. Natural events could be deemed the outcome of acts of the immortals' love-making, rivalries, and battles. Just as children at an early developmental stage believe that their parents can influence nature, so prescientific man believed that his kings and priests had special influence with these deities.

In anthropomorphizing nature, man everywhere endowed it with the emotions, drives, desires, and conflicts he knew existed in himself and other persons; and he gradually elaborated these attributions of human characteristics to nature into tales about his gods and about ancestral heroes who had been close to the gods and had protected his forebears in battles against the dragons and giants representative of adverse natural forces. Mythopoesis categorizes together events that otherwise seem unrelated and disparate—for example, connecting the winter solstice to regicide through myths of the slaying of the old king, symbolic of the dying year, by his supplanter; or associating the coming of spring with marriage through a ritual in which a selected youth copulated with the May Queen to assure the fertility of the land. Categorization that bestows a type of equivalence to man and some aspect of nature is essential to efforts to influence nature by ritual, magic, or prayer, and thereby to lessen feelings of helplessness before the contingencies of nature.

Thus, in developing myths that sought to explain the rituals used to cope with natural phenomena, man told tales about the wellsprings of human behavior. Myths came to have much to say about human nature in terms of the motives, passions, and perverse inclinations that led deities and heroes representative of nature to act as they did. Further, man had to live with human nature, which was even more unpredictable than other natural phenomena and contained sources of catastrophe. He sought to understand the forces that welled up within himself and disrupted his intentions and his ability to live together with his fellows cooperatively. Therefore, while myths concern the power of nature over man, they also concern the power of nature *within* him, to which he so often wishes to give way but which he has learned he must hold in check lest it overpower and destroy him.

One means of keeping human behavior within the limits required for social living was the development of myths that told not only of the awesome or dreadful deeds carried out by heroic progenitors, but also of the torments they suffered as consequences of their acts. Although the awful deed may have originally been a ritual act that was considered pious and proper—such as Tantalus' sacrifice of his son Pelops, whom he fed to the Olympians—as myth became divorced from ritual and as the progress of civilization made such acts abhorrent to people, the myth changed to tell of the punishments that befell the perpetrator of the act. Tantalus came to suffer perpetual torment in Hades and his descendants were fated to sin and suffer even unto the fifth generation.

The myth can thus serve as a major defense of the cultural superego, a means of reinforcing a basic taboo, by holding before the people what befell a godlike ancestor when he committed an "unnatural" act or gave way to a forbidden impulsion—forbidden because it endangered the stability of the social order and the proper development of the individual. Because the family forms the primary unit of every society, many of the most telling myths concern the devastating consequences of breaches of intrafamilial bonds.

Let us consider very briefly the myths of Tantalus and his descendants that led to the curse upon the House of Agamemnon, the topic of tragedies by Aeschylus, Sophocles, and Euripides. Tantalus fed his son Pelops to the Olympians. Pelops, whom the gods reconstructed, gained his bride Hip-

podamia and her father's kingdom by plotting with her to kill
her father. His sons, Atreus and Thyestes, fought and cheated
each other for possession of Queen Aerope, and when Thyestes
took Aerope from him, Atreus fed Thyestes' sons to him as a
stew. Aegisthus, who was both Thyestes' son and his grandson
(Thyestes had raped his own daughter), not only killed Atreus
to avenge his father and brothers, but also later killed Atreus'
son, Agamemnon. Aegisthus was helped by Agamemnon's wife
Clytemnestra, who was embittered because Agamemnon had
sacrificed their daughter, Iphigenia, to the gods. Orestes, the
son of Agamemnon and Clytemnestra, was then placed in the
hapless situation of being obligated to commit matricide to
avenge his father.[1]

Or, let us leave Mycenae and move to Thebes and the
House of Cadmus, to review the misfortunes that beset
Oedipus and his offspring. The troubles did not arise just
because Oedipus had carried out the forbidden heroic fantasy
of childhood and killed his father and procreated with his
mother—thus breaking two of the fundamental taboos of
society. His father, Laius, who was homosexual, feared to sleep
with his queen, Jocasta. When she tricked him into having
intercourse and later gave birth to Oedipus, Laius feared that
his son would kill him. Then, to placate her husband, Jocasta
agreed to commit infanticide by exposing Oedipus. Oedipus,
not having been raised by his parents, had no reason to
recognize, respect, or fear his father, or to be inhibited from
sleeping with the woman he did not know was his mother. The
misfortunes of the House of Cadmus did not end with
Oedipus. His sons slew one another in a war of succession; his
daughter Antigone was entombed alive for defying the order of
her uncle, Creon, by carrying out burial rites for one of her

1. For a more complete discussion of this sequence of myths and their ritual
significance, and also those of the House of Cadmus, see T. Lidz, *Hamlet's Enemy*.

brothers. The punishment of Antigone, in turn, brought tragedy upon Creon through the suicide of his son Haemon, Antigone's fiancé.

The force of such myths in bolstering a cultural superego was recognized and emphasized by the great classic dramatists, who used these myths to carry their audiences to the very core of the human dilemma, and to hold before mankind the dread penalties that come from infractions of sacred family obligations. Aeschylus, for example, utilized the Orestes myth not only to consider how the stability of the state and of the family depended upon father-right becoming equal to mother-right, but also to hold before his compatriots the need to replace the code of family vengeance, which could only breed havoc from generation to generation and disrupt the unity of the city-state, with civic law and trial by jury. Aeschylus could cap his great trilogy about the House of Agamemnon by having Athena proclaim her timeless commandment, "Let no man live, / Uncurbed by law nor curbed by tyranny."

It is apparent that many of the fundamental ethical principles conveyed by myth are not simply products of superstition. The basic problems that require resolution have been much the same in all societies: how to curb the aggressive and sexual drives that so easily disrupt any social system, but especially how to control intrafamilial murder and incest in order to permit the development of the stable family, which everywhere forms the basis for communal living. Fathers, mothers, sons, and daughters must be able to live together despite the passions that arise among them because of the needs, loves, jealousies, and hatreds they have for one another.

Mythic thought—in contrast to science, which seeks new knowledge and new techniques wherever they may lead— gains insights and directives for living from the cyclic phenomena of life, phenomena that recur from season to season, from life to life, from parent to children, and even from civilization to civilization. Myth is concerned with experiences that recur because they are inherent in the human condition —the cycle of life, the rivalries between fathers and sons, the jealousies of siblings, the displacement of each generation by the next, the incompleteness of each sex, the eternal desire for closeness, the fear of engulfment by mothers—the repetitive, timeless themes symbolized in the myths of Oedipus, Orestes, Hamlet, Antigone, Persephone. Here, insight and wisdom are sought through the diffuse tale that symbolically encompasses events of countless lives, all different and yet ever the same in essentials; always old and still ever new, as new times, customs, and listeners give it new meaning. It is a use of intellect that is different from that of scientific thinking—but a use of intellect that has room for unconscious sources of knowledge, with the ambivalence and the conflicted drives and emotions that are of the essence in human affairs. We may do well to pay heed to what the mythical seeks to convey, for it can lead not only to deeper knowledge of human behavior but perhaps even to the wisdom needed to direct human affairs—wisdom that the customary ways of pursuing science have been unable to provide because they contain no room for values.

When we consider the behavioral and social sciences, including psychodynamic or psychoanalytic psychology, we find that following the model of the physical sciences and eliminating ethical values often renders the field sterile. We are concerned with value judgments that have ethical connotations for at least two reasons: because we are interested in the maintenance and improvement of the social systems that man requires as a social animal who is dependent upon the assimilation of cultural techniques and societal roles, and who must collaborate with others to survive; and because we seek through the behavioral sciences to promote the well-being of individuals.

Man's need to construct ethical principles and adhere to them has often been ascribed to the need to maintain the society upon which he depends. Durkheim (1925) considered that the function of morality is to link the individual to one or more groups, and that it is devised for society, by society. "If a society is the end of morality," he wrote, "it [morality] is also its product." He considered that the foundations of morality had to be established in the schools, where rules could be and must be enforced. He considered the family unsuited for fostering morality, maintaining, "Because the family is closer to the individual, it provides less impersonal—and hence, less lofty goals. The circle of family interests is so restricted that it is in large measure the same as individual interests" (Durkheim, 1925, p. 74). I shall take exception to both of his arguments, and hold that ethics are essential to the integration of the individual as well as for society; and that although the school can be very important, the foundations of a person's morality are laid down within the family.[2]

Psychoanalysis has focused attention upon superego formation as the person's means of internalizing parental directives and containing aggressive and sexual impulsions. Although Freud originally considered the development of the superego in terms of a transformation of libidinal energy released by the resolution of the child's Oedipal attachment to the mother, he later emphasized that the superego is, so to speak, a precipitate of prolonged parental influence upon the child, and that the parent's influence includes not only "the personalities of the actual parents but also the family, racial and national traditions handed on through them, as well as the demands of the immediate social *milieu* which they represent." Further, he notes that a person's superego also "receives contributions

2. I shall not here consider Piaget's emphasis on the role of peer groups in promoting a "morality of cooperation" in the older child; but Piaget also tends to neglect the family's role in fostering a morality of cooperation as well as a morality of constraint. See J. Piaget, *The Moral Judgment of the Child*, particularly his discussion of Durkheim's concepts in chapter 4, "The Two Moralities of the Child and Types of Social Relations."

from later successors and substitutes of his parents, such as teachers and models in public life of admired social ideals" (Freud, 1940, p. 146).

It has become apparent that the nature of a person's superego depends not only upon the personalities of both parents but also upon how they relate to one another, as well as to the child. However, the superego is important not only for the society and the person's relationship to the society in which he lives, but also for the integrated development of the individual. The superego, by providing inner guidance and helping with the containment of id impulses, permits the establishment of adequate boundaries between the self and the parents, enables individuation within the family and from the family, and fosters growth through identification with, and internalization of, parental figures. Stated succinctly, the opposite side of the society's need to socialize the child is the child's need for socialization, enculturation, and delimitation. Those who would carry to an extreme Freud's notion of society as the source of repressions that cause neuroses, without regard for his recognition of man's dependence upon society, and who therefore wish to free the child from all restrictive forces, fail to understand the importance of internalized parental and societal delimitation to coherent personality organization.

An understanding of the nature and importance of the superego—or if you will, of the conscience—leads one to give the family a cardinal role in the individual's ethical development. However, various aspects of family life other than superego formation influence a person's ethics. Durkheim, as I have noted, argued that because family interests are in large measure the same as individual interests, they cannot foster the child's moral development. In contrast, I believe that precisely for such reasons it is within the family that the child learns that the interests of others, and of the group upon which he depends, can be as important as, if not more important than, his own wishes and even his own needs. In the family, ethical principles have a real and concrete meaning. Here, self-interest is not very different from the interests of others and of the family group as a whole; here one's own happiness is bound to that of others whom one loves or seeks to love, even when one hates them and when their lack of affection breeds despair and anger (Lidz, 1963).

The infant first relinquishes his demand for immediate gratification of needs for the reward of having a more relaxed mother. The prolonged helplessness of the child requires that he be raised by persons to whom his welfare is as important as, if not more important than, their own. If, as Erik Erikson (1950) has emphasized, the child's fundamental needs are not met when he is unable to care for himself and is only aware of them in terms of diffuse discomfort, he will lack a basic trust that influences all later relationships. Then, if his mother cannot foster the child's individuation from his initial symbiosis with her, the child can never become self-sufficient enough to consider the well-being of others. Then, too, if the father, jealous of the time and attention his wife pays to the child, becomes hostile to the child, the child is apt to build up patterns of counteraggression very early in life.

I cannot here continue to enumerate other such specific familial influences upon the child's ethical development. Beyond such factors, the family is a true small group in which the behavior of any family member affects all, and in which reciprocally interrelating roles must be found or the personality of one or more members will be distorted. Here, children learn to place the welfare of the collectivity above their own because the security provided by the family is of paramount importance to them. Children gain their earliest directives for relating to others more from the behavior of parents than from what they teach; and what the parents admire in each other enters into the child's ego ideal along with the parents' expectations and hopes for the child. Disgrace of parents brings shame to the child; and disillusionment with them is the usual precursor of disillusionment with the world and alienation from society.

In general, a child will feel secure and will trust others if his parents have placed his needs on the same level as their own and those of his siblings. He will become prone to hate or to do violence if subjected to arbitrary punishments; and he is apt to become devious and dishonest if he can gain his needs only through circumvention. The child emulates who the parents are rather than what they pretend to be. The ethical principles that a child gains in his family—which can also be unethical principles—do not depend so much upon precepts or punishments as upon the parents' characters, the nature of the home they provide, and how much of themselves they can give to those who need them and depend upon them.

Further, the family is the basic social system in all societies, the first group in which a person lives, and the group that is treated as the primary unit of society; the well-being of both the individual and the society depends greatly upon the stability and integrity of the family as a unit. It is in the family of origin that the child learns to value or devalue such institutions as the family, marriage, and parenthood; learns the reliability or arbitrariness of authority, and whether power and authority lead to responsibility or self-gratification; learns the worth of collaboration or the need always to consider one's own welfare first. In general, it is a child's experiences with his family's transactions that largely determine how he will relate to social systems and evaluate the worth of social institutions in general.

More than the ethics of individuals is involved: the stability of the family is related to the continuity of the ethos of the society. The provision of a secure family milieu has, however, become more difficult as nuclear families have become isolated from kin, as the value of tradition as a source of guidance has diminished, as marriages have increasingly occurred between persons of different cultural backgrounds, as male and female

roles have become less definite, as parents have less preparation for parenthood before marriage, as less of the mother's
lifespan has been spent in the home and in mothering. We
place great demands upon the persons who become parents
and organize a family, and the strain upon parents becomes
greater as they come to appreciate how greatly the child's
well-being and his future as an adult depend upon how and in
what setting he is raised. We place great demands and provide
little guidance and support, as if we still believed that the
capacity to be a parent is essentially inborn.

It is at such times, when people turn from tradition as a
guide for living, when the value of ethical principles is
doubted, when many decisions rest upon individual choice,
that cultures start to crumble. If the child's emotional needs
are unsatisfied in his family of origin, he later requires more
from a marriage than can be provided by a spouse. If the
family offers less to the child, he is less willing to sacrifice for
his own family when an adult. When the security and pleasure
that derive from close interpersonal relationships begin to fail,
a people turns to narcissistic gratification and hedonistic
choices. Marriages become less stable and the responsibilities
of parenthood are avoided. The family, which forms the
matrix of society and is the basic carrier of tradition, declines.
If, as I believe, the decline of civilization can follow upon the
deterioration of its family life, it becomes apparent that man's
ways of adaptation are intimately related to his ethics.

I have sought to clarify the relationships between the family,
myth, and ethics in response to a new challenge that confronts
our society—a challenge that arises from the realization that
what a person becomes depends greatly upon the emotional,
cultural, social, and cognitive milieu in which he is raised.

In closing, I wish to reemphasize several issues:

1. Whereas ethical principles are relative, varying from
society to society, certain basic issues are common to societies

everywhere and similar prohibitions and imperatives are reflected in very different mythologies. They are common to different cultures because they concern the preservation and stability of the family that everywhere forms the nexus of society.

2. Ethical principles not only are essential to preserve the society man requires, but also are essential to preserve the integration and stability of the individual.

3. The family not only teaches and imposes a "morality of constraint," but also provides the basis for a "morality of cooperation," because within the family the well-being of the individual is intimately bound up with the good of the family as a unit.

4. The taming and control of primitive passions and narcissistic strivings rest not only upon a constraining super-ego, cultural taboos, and legal edicts, but also upon the family as a developmental milieu that promotes the harmonious development of offspring and fosters understanding and collaboration rather than the intensification of intrafamilial rivalries and erotic attractions.

5. When science is applied to human affairs, values cannot be excluded, particularly when we seek to foster emotional stability. Ethical issues related to family life have pertinence to mental health and its transmission from generation to generation.

6. Myth, with its emphasis upon the recurrent in human affairs, has served to foster and to preserve ethical principles essential to the integration and well-being of the individual, as well as to the stability of society.

REFERENCES

Butler, S. *Erewhon* (1872). New York: Modern Library, 1927.
Durkheim, E. *Moral Education* (1925). New York: Free Press of Glencoe, 1961.

Erikson, E. *Childhood and Society*. New York: W. W. Norton, 1950.

Freud, S. *Civilization and its Discontents* (1930). In *The Standard Edition of the Complete Psychological Works of Sigmund Freud*, vol. 21. London: Hogarth Press, 1961.

————. *An Outline of Psycho-Analysis* (1940). In *The Standard Edition of the Complete Psychological Works of Sigmund Freud*, vol. 23. London: Hogarth Press, 1964.

Lidz, T. *The Family and Human Adaptation*; New York: International Universities Press, 1963.

————. "The Family: The Source of Human Resources." In *Human Resources and Economic Welfare. Essays in Honor of Eli Ginzberg*, ed. I. Berg. New York: Columbia University Press, 1972.

————. *Hamlet's Enemy*. New York: Basic Books, 1975.

Piaget, J. *The Child's Conception of the World*. Paterson, N.J.: Littlefield, Adams, 1929.

————. *The Moral Judgment of the Child*. Glencoe, Ill.: Free Press, 1948.

9

Healing through Meeting:
A Dialogical Approach to Psychotherapy
and Family Therapy

Maurice Friedman

In the spring of 1957, Martin Buber came from Jerusalem to Washington, D.C. to deliver the Fourth William Alanson White Memorial Lectures on the subject "The Contribution of Philosophical Anthropology to Psychology," and also to conduct a seminar for thirty of us on dreams and the unconscious. During that same spring I was teaching a public course on comparative religion and psychotherapy at the Washington School of Psychiatry and a private seminar on the problem of evil for a handful of the faculty. The latter seminar was held at the home of Edith and Oscar Weigert in Chevy Chase and was attended by Leslie Farber, Margaret Rioch, Ben Weininger, the Weigerts, and myself, and once in a while by Buber too. It was also during this spring that I moderated the dialogue between Martin Buber and Carl Rogers at a conference centered around Buber at the University of Michigan. Looking back, seventeen years later, I am impressed by the many seeds of "healing through meeting" that were sown in my own life and in those of others by the events of that spring. I can think of no more fitting tribute to Edith Weigert on her eightieth birthday than to write on this theme.

One aspect of the movement of existential psychology and psychiatry that has consistently been neglected, even if touched on here and there, is that of healing through meeting. Though it has been present as a minor theme in much of the literature, a strong light has never been trained on it so as to bring out its true importance and to illuminate the issues and problems that it raises. All therapy relies to a greater or lesser extent on the meeting between therapist and client and the meeting among clients. But only a few theories have singled out meeting—the sphere of the "between"—as the central, as opposed to ancillary, source of healing.

From the very beginning of formal psychoanalysis, healing through meeting was already built into the system as an indispensable means to the end of overcoming fixation and repressions. Even if the therapeutic situation was toned down by Freud's asking the patient to lie on the couch rather than face him, it still was a meeting—in contrast, say, to the situation in which a psychologist administers a Rorschach or a TAT test. Freudian theory, to be sure, sees the ego as the servant of three masters—the superego, the id, and the environment. "Freud fought against his humanistic personal urges through his 'scientism,' " writes Ivan Boszormenyi-Nagy, "and he abhorred Ferenczi's relational emphasis on therapeutic method." [1]

Yet we cannot imagine Freud working year after year with people and dealing with them only as objects. When we turn to Carl Jung, whose theory is even more preoccupied with the intrapsychic than Freud's, it is startling to realize the extent to which his therapy is centered on the dimension of meeting, or dialogue. In *The Undiscovered Self* Jung says, "All over the world, it is being recognized today that what is being treated is not a symptom, but a patient." [2] The more the doctor schematizes, the more the patient quite rightly resists. The

1. Letter from Nagy to Maurice Friedman, June 21, 1974.
2. C. G. Jung, *The Undiscovered Self*, trans. R. F. C. Hull (Boston: Little, Brown & Co., 1958), p. 12.

patient demands to be dealt with in his or her uniqueness, and not just as part of a problem, and to do this the therapist must engage and risk himself as a person.

Healing through meeting is not restricted to psychotherapy. The great surgeon does not just deal with an anatomy; he deals with an actual person, and he has to know when and how to deal with this person. The same applies to the whole process of dying, which is absorbing the interest of so many today. The way in which people have been left to deal by themselves with their problems of dying, as if there were no problems, has represented a great avoidance of the reality of meeting, especially by doctors and nurses. A moving contrast can be seen in the approaches of two sisters whom I know, both of whom are psychiatrists and both of whom work with people who are dying—one with children, the other with older cancer patients. As an example of the work of both, the first sister told me of how she encouraged the dying children to communicate with her through painting and of one child who painted a ship and said, "This is a ship that's going out. This is me." The recognition by the child of the fact that he was going to die and the therapist's simple acceptance of what he shared with her were meaningful events that deserve to be called healing through meeting. A recent conference on death was aptly subtitled "A Dialogue with the Living," for death is a concern not of the dead but of the living. The persistent refusal to face the reality of dying in our culture has made meeting very difficult. No two people, even in the prime of their lives, can really meet except through the acceptance by both of the reality of death, of aloneness, of that "lonesome valley" that you've got to go to by yourself.[3]

Another very important development in our time is the

3. See Maurice Friedman, *The Hidden Human Image* (New York: Delacorte Press [hardback] and Delta Books [paperback], 1974), chap. 9, "Death and the Dialogue with the Absurd."

meeting between the therapist and the psychotherapy group
and among the members of the group. Moreover, as much as
the term *meeting* is distorted by the way in which *encounter* is
used today, the whole encounter movement has within it the
seed of the happening between and among people.

I have taken the phrase "healing through meeting" from
the title which Martin Buber gave to the posthumous book by
the Swiss psychoanalyst Hans Trüb *(Heilung aus der Begegnung)*.
As long as there has been society, something recognizable as
healing through meeting has taken place. The parent, the
teacher, the nurse, the shaman, the medicine man—anyone
who lays hands on another or helps another—is involved in
healing through meeting. Very often, as among the Shakers
and the Quakers, the spirit comes and moves in the midst of a
group of people: we cannot say in such cases that it proceeds
from any one person, or even from the combination of the
"spirituality" of the "healer" and the "faith" of the healed. In
one seventeenth-century Friends meeting in England, a "possessed" woman was healed by the whole meeting and not by
any one person appointed to the task or endowed with
charismatic power.

The fundamental fact of human existence is the meeting, or
dialogue, between man and man. The psychological, the
psychic stream of happenings within each man, is only the
accompaniment of the dialogical. It is not itself the reality and
goal of human existence. Even individuation is not the goal
but only the indispensable way to the goal—a fact insuf-
ficiently recognized by those psychotherapists and psychologists who see the importance of mutual relations largely as the
function of the individual's becoming—namely, as a means to
the end of health, maturity, or integration. The basis of man's
life with man, as Buber points out in *The Knowledge of Man*,[4] is

---

4. Martin Buber, *The Knowledge of Man. A Philosophy of the Interhuman*, ed. with an
introductory essay (chap. 1) by Maurice Friedman (New York: Harper Torchbooks,
1966), chap. 2, "Distance and Relation."

the capacity of each person to confirm the other in what he is and can become. This mutual confirmation of men is most fully realized in making the other present—imagining quite concretely what another person is wishing, feeling, perceiving, and thinking. It is through this making present that I grasp another as a self, an event which is only complete when he *knows* himself made present by me in his wholeness, unity, and uniqueness. It is this event of making present which induces the other's inmost self-becoming and not, as people tend to think today, his relationship to himself. If I overlook the real "otherness" of the other person, I shall not be able to help him, for I shall see him in my own image or in terms of my ready-made categories.

Real healing is only possible through mutuality, trust, and partnership in a common situation. If the psychotherapist is content to "analyze" the patient, writes Buber, "to bring to light unknown factors from his microcosm, and to set to some conscious work in life the energies which have been transformed by such an emergence, . . . he may help a soul which is diffused and poor in structure to collect and order itself to some extent. But the real matter, the regeneration of an atrophied personal center, will not be achieved. This can only be done by one who grasps the buried latent unity of the suffering soul . . . in the person-to-person attitude of a partner, not by the consideration and examination of an object." This common situation does not exclude the difference of role and function determined by the very difference of purpose which led each to enter the relationship. "The specific 'healing' relation would come to an end the moment the patient thought of, and succeeded in practicing 'inclusion' and experiencing the event from the doctor's pole as well." [5]

The therapist must try to overcome the unconscious imposi-

5. Martin Buber, *I and Thou*, 2d rev. ed. with postscript by author added, trans. Ronald Gregor Smith (New York: Chas. Scribner's Sons, 1958), pp. 132–34.

tion of the categories of his school on the patient through "obedient listening"—that is, using the whole force of his being to leave the patient to himself. "The real master responds to uniqueness." The therapist's openness and willingness to receive whatever comes is necessary in order that the patient may trust existentially and give himself up into the hands of the therapist so that contact may arise between them. In existential healing the therapist perceives and confirms the personal direction of the patient that lies hidden in the present. In the strongest illness that appears in the life of a person, the highest potentiality of this person may be manifesting itself in negative form. Healing does not mean bringing up the old, but shaping the new: it is not confirming the negative, but counterbalancing with the positive.[6]

One of the most important issues that the concept of healing through meeting raises is the extent to which healing proceeds from a specific healer—priest, sorcerer, shaman, or therapist— and the extent to which healing takes place in the "between" —in the relationship between therapist and client, among the members of a group or family, or even in a community. When the latter is the case, is there a special role, nonetheless, for the therapist as facilitator, midwife, enabler, or partner in a "dialogue of touchstones"? We must also ask whether such healing takes place through an existential grace which cannot be planned and counted on, however much it can be helped along. To what extent does healing through meeting imply that meeting must also be the *goal* as well as the means to that goal? And to what extent are we talking about a two-sided event that is not susceptible to techniques in the sense of willing and manipulating in order to bring about a certain result?

6. Based on "The Unconscious," notes taken by Maurice Friedman at three sessions of a seminar given by Martin Buber for the Washington (D.C.) School of Psychiatry (1957), published in Martin Buber, *A Believing Humanism: Gleanings*, ed. and trans. with an introduction and explanatory comments by Maurice Friedman (New York: Simon & Schuster Paperbacks, 1969), pp. 152–73.

Another important problem that healing through meeting raises is that of the limits of responsibility of the helper. To what extent does the therapist have an ego involvement such that he feels himself a success if the patient is healed or a failure if he is not? A therapist open to the new vistas of healing through meeting will feel that more is demanded of him than his professional methods and his professional role, that "abyss calls to abyss," as Buber puts it in the essay "Healing through Meeting" that he wrote as a preface to Trüb's book—not to the technical superiority of the therapist but to his actual self. In his book *Power and Innocence*,[7] Rollo May tells of a black woman patient who felt so powerless and so cut off from her own anger that May had to become angry for her. But he added, "I did not do this just as a technique. I really became angry." Only through his real personal involvement was the woman able to find access to her anger.

What is crucial is not the skill of the therapist but what takes place *between* the therapist and the client and between the client and other people. No amount of therapy can be of decisive help if a person is too enmeshed in a family, community, or culture in which the seeds of healing are constantly choked off and the attempts at restoration of personal wholeness are thwarted by the destructive elements built into the system itself. One of the great violations of reality that psychotherapy has often been guilty of in our age is that it has focused so much on the inner psychic world—the neurosis or the complex of the person—that parents, family, and culture have been treated as psychic symbols rather than as the concrete social context of the person's day-to-day existence. In Jungian therapy the other often tends to be regarded as the "anima" or the "animus," the feminine or the masculine figure, or the projected "shadow," rather than as

7. Rollo May, *Power and Innocence. a search for the Sources of Violence* (New York: W. W. Norton & Co., 1972).

someone of unique value in his or her otherness. In much Freudian therapy, not to mention that popular Freudianism which has such a strong hold on our culture, it is the same.

That psychotherapist who above all others made his lifework and his way of life that of healing through meeting is the late Swiss psychiatrist Hans Trüb. In an essay on "Individuation, Guilt, and Decision," Trüb describes how he went through a decade-long crisis in which he broke with his personal and doctrinal dependence on Jung in favor of the new insights that arose through his friendship with Martin Buber. What had the greatest influence on Trüb was not Buber's doctrine but the meeting with him person to person, and it is from this meeting that the revolutionary change in Trüb's method of psychotherapy proceeded.[8] Put in terms of the image of man, we could say that it was not the image of man that Buber consciously presented in his writings and speaking which influenced Trüb, but the image of man that Buber communicated in his dialogue with Trüb—an image, therefore, that was made up of the basic attitudes of both men and the dialogue between them, rather than one possessing any visual form or conceptual content.

Trüb writes that in time he found himself fully disarmed by the fact that in conversation Buber was not concerned about the ideas of his partner but about the partner himself. It became ever clearer to Trüb that in such unreserved inter-change it is simply not possible to bring any hidden intention with one and to pursue it. In this dialogue one individuality did not triumph over the other, for each remained continually the same. Yet Trüb emerged from this meeting " 'renewed for all time,' with my knowledge of the reality of things brought

8. Hans Trüb, "Individuation, Schuld und Entscheidung. Über die Grenzen der Psychologie," in *Die kulturelle Bedeutung der Komplexen Psychologie*, ed. Psychologischen Club Zürich (Berlin: Julius Spring Verlag, 1935), pp. 529–42, 553.

one step nearer to the truth." Particularly important for Trüb seems to have been Buber's practice of "inclusion," or experiencing the other side, which Trüb describes as letting a soft tone sound and swell in himself and listening for the echo from the other side.[9]

Trüb describes how in his work with his patients he became aware of the invariable tendency of the primary consciousness to become monological and self-defeating. He also tells how this closed circle of the self was again and again forced outward toward relationship through those times when, despite his will, he found himself confronting his patient not as an analyst but as human being to human being. From these experiences he came to understand the full meaning of the analyst's responsibility. The analyst takes responsibility for lost and forgotten things, and with the aid of his psychology he helps to bring them to light. But he knows in the depths of his self that the secret meaning of these things that have been brought to consciousness first reveals itself *in the outgoing to the other*.[10]

> *Psychology* as science and *psychology* as function know about the soul of man as about something in the third person. . . . They look down from above into the world of inner things, into the inner world of the individual. And they deal with its contents as with their "objects." They give names and they create classifications while carefully investigating the manifold connections and presenting them vividly in meaningful systems.
>
> But the psychotherapist in his work with the ill is *essentially a human being*. . . . Therefore he seeks and loves the human being in his patients and allows it . . . to come to him ever again.[11]

9. Ibid., p. 554.
10. Ibid., pp. 543–50.
11. Hans Trüb, "Individuation, Guilt, and Decision" (selection) in *The Worlds of Existentialism*, ed. with introductions and a conclusion by Maurice Friedman (New

The personal experience which caused Trüb to move from the dialectical psychology of Jung to the dialogical anthropology of Buber was, he tells us, an overwhelming sense of guilt. This guilt was no longer such as could be explained away or removed, for it was subjectively experienced as the guilt of a person who had stepped out of real relationship to the world and tried to live in a spiritual world above reality. Trüb, like Buber, holds that guilt is an essential factor in a person's relations with others and that it performs the necessary function of leading him to desire to set these relations right. It is just here, in the real guilt of the person who has not responded to the legitimate claim and address of the world, that the possibility of transformation and healing lies. This is so because true guilt, in contrast to neurotic guilt, takes place *between* man and man. It is an ontological reality of which the feeling of guilt is only the subjective and psychological counterpart. For this reason Buber says that guilt does not reside in the person but that the person stands, in the most realistic sense, in the guilt that envelops him.

Similarly, the repression of guilt and the neuroses resulting from this repression are not merely psychological phenomena but real events between men. Therefore, the man who is sick from existential guilt must follow a path made up of three stages in order to be healed, Buber holds. First, he must illuminate his guilt by recognizing that, however different he may be now, he is the person who took this burden of guilt on himself; second, he must persevere in this illumination; and third, he must repair the injured order of the world, either with the person he wronged or by establishing a new dialogical relation at some other point. In T. S. Eliot's *The Cocktail Party*, Sir Henry Harcourt-Reilly tells Edward that he must learn to live with his guilt but that there is nothing he can do about it

York: Random House, 1964; Chicago: The University of Chicago Press and Phoenix Books [paperback], 1973), p. 497.

in relation to the person toward whom he is guilty. Buber, in contrast, holds that guilt means a rupture of the dialogical relationship, an injury of the existential order of "the common," and as such must be repaired by again entering into dialogue with that person or with the world.[12]

Real guilt is the beginning of *ethos,* or responsibility, writes Trüb in his essay "From Self to World," [13] but before the patient can become aware of it, he must be helped by the analyst to become aware of himself in general. This the analyst does through playing the part both of confidante and big brother. He gives the neurotic the understanding that the world has denied him and makes it more and more possible for him to step out of his self-imprisonment and into a genuine relation with the analyst. In doing this, says Trüb, the analyst must avoid both the intimacy of a private I-Thou relationship with the patient *and* the temptation of dealing with the patient as an object. This means, in effect, that he must have just that dialogical relationship of concrete but one-sided inclusion on which Buber insisted in his postscript to *I and Thou*: it cannot become the mutual inclusion of friendship without destroying the therapeutic possibilities of the relationship; but neither can it make the patient into an It. The analyst must be able to risk himself and to participate in the process of individuation.

The analyst must see the illness of the patient as an illness of his relations with the world, writes Trüb. The roots of the neurosis lie both in the patient's closing himself off from the world and in the pattern of society itself and its rejection and nonconfirmation of the patient. Consequently, the analyst must change at some point from the consoler who takes the part of the patient against the world, to the person who puts before the patient the claim of the world. This change is

12. Martin Buber, *The Knowledge of Man*, chap. 6, "Guilt and Guilt Feelings," trans. Maurice Friedman. Cf. Hans Trüb, "Individuation, Schuld und Entscheidung," pp. 531-39.

13. Hans Trüb, "Vom Selbst zur Welt," *Psyche* 1 (1947): 41-67.

necessary to complete the second part of the cure—that establishment of real relationship with the world which can only take place in the world itself. On the analyst falls the task of preparing the way for the resumption in direct meeting of the interrupted dialogical relationship between the individual and the community. The psychotherapist must test the patient's finding of himself by the criterion of whether his self-realization can be the starting point for a new personal meeting with the world. The patient must go forth whole in himself, but he must also recognize that it is not his own self but the world with which he must be concerned. This does not mean, however, that the patient is simply integrated with or adjusted to the world. He does not cease to be a real person, responsible for himself, but at the same time he enters into a responsible relationship with his community.[14]

In *Healing through Meeting*, Trüb states his approach to psychotherapy through a systematic confrontation with the psychology of Jung. Man's self, the center of his personality, becomes actualized only as he discloses himself as a partner to the world; and so, too, the living sense of psychic processes, both healthy and pathological, is revealed only from this self-disclosure. Therefore, to know his patient the psychotherapist must recognize him in his partnership with the world. To do this an objective knowledge is not enough. The therapist must experience the patient as a partner in his own meeting with him. It is through this eye-to-eye confrontation that the patient's capacity for meeting begins to be restored.

By viewing the isolated patient from the beginning as one who has sacrificed his capacity for dialogue in withdrawing his self from meeting with the world, and by addressing him immediately, anthropological psychotherapy sets him up as a fellow human being, a Thou, the

14. *The Worlds of Existentialism*, pp. 497–99.

original partner in a fully human meeting. It seeks out
this stubborn self, this introvert captive of the psyche, and
will not release it. It summons this self by name as the one
called upon to answer, the one personally responsible.
And by addressing it in this manner, it challenges the self
to disclose itself in its self and to individuate itself in the
new dialogue with the physician-partner and beyond him
in intercourse—and not merely the introverted kind—
with the world.[15]

For Trüb the dialogical meeting is both the starting point
and the goal of therapy. The success or failure of the cure
focuses in the risk of this meeting. The tension of psychic
conflict that derives from the contradiction of the conscious
and unconscious arrives at a psychotherapeutic resolution in
the framework of this basic partnership relation. "The healing
process takes place between *this* physician and *this* patient, in
the totality of their personal confrontation." [16] The therapist
embodies for the patient a loving inclination of the world
which seeks to restore the patient's dispirited and mistrustful
self to a new dialogical meeting with the forces of nature and
history. Thus the therapist quiets and harmonizes the psychic
tension of the patient, not only according to the latter's wish,
but as a partner penetrating the personal basis of his being, the
actual origin of that elemental introversion which nourishes all
neurosis. The unconscious is precisely the personal element
that is lost in the course of development, that escapes
consciousness. In dealing with this lost element, the psychotherapist cannot point to a truth which he *has* but only to a
truth to be sought *between* him and the patient. Only thus can
he again equalize the enormous advantage given him by the
fact that the other one seeks him out and asks for help in his
need. Thus the equality of respect for which the humanistic

15. Ibid., pp. 500–01.
16. Ibid., p. 502.

psychologist seeks is attained, according to Trüb, not by the insistence on a complete mutuality of situation, but by the recognition of the *betweenness* itself as the place where real meeting, real healing, and real finding take place.

It is very important, of course, that the therapist not place the demand for responsibility in dialogue upon the patient before he is ready for it. That is why the reconstruction of the capacity for dialogue must go hand in hand with the methodical attempt to loosen and dismantle the complex defense mechanisms in the psychic realm of expression as fast as the recuperating self permits. "Without this supplemental assistance of depth psychology, what is dialogically expected of the patient's self in the meeting situation with the world would place too great a demand on it and expose it to the danger of regression." [17]

But Trüb does *not* hold, like Jung and his followers, that one must first become individuated and only then enter into dialogue with other men. The therapist, says Trüb, must keep in view "the one true goal of healing, the unlocking of the locked up person for the meeting with the world." [18] Only this enables him to answer *both* for the patient *and* for the world. Only by so doing can the therapist risk personal commitment, even to the neurotic self-entanglement of the patient. Only starting from the meeting as partner can physician and patient hold their ground with a positive attitude in the face of the cure's completion, which generally occurs unexpectedly and which may be compared, Trüb suggests, to a leap over an abyss. All this implies no choice between the inner, personal wholeness and the social self, such as Jung makes in his repeated valuation of the former above the latter. On the contrary, "the willingness of the self to meet the world, the situation of a living dialogue, that is between 'within' and

17. Ibid.
18. Ibid., p. 503.

'without,' should be striven for and furthered *simultaneously* with the effort to attain a psychic integration of the self." [19] When the psychological cooperation and dialectical interaction of patient and therapist is conducted dialogically, with mutual personal trust between therapist and patient, then there gradually awakens and grows in the patient at one and the same time, and as corollaries of the same happening, a new confidence in himself *and* in the other.[20]

It is to Hans Trüb that Buber points in "Healing through Meeting," as the man who broke the trail as a practicing psychotherapist in the recognition and realization of the therapeutic possibilities of dialogue. Speaking of the crisis through which the psychotherapist passes when he discovers the paradox of his vocation, Buber writes:

> In a decisive hour, together with the patient entrusted to and trusting in him, he has left the closed room of psychological treatment in which the analyst rules by means of his systematic and methodological superiority and has stepped forth with him into the air of the world where self is exposed to self. There, in the closed room where one probed and treated the isolated psyche according to the inclination of the self-encapsulated patient, the patient was referred to ever-deeper levels of his inwardness as to his proper world; here outside, in the immediacy of one human standing over against another, the encapsulation must and can be broken through, and a transformed, healed relationship must and can be opened to the person who is sick in his relationship to otherness— to the world of the other which he cannot remove into his

19. Ibid.

20. Ibid., pp. 504–05. These selections are the only published translations in English of Hans Trüb, *Heilung aus der begegnung. Eine Auseinandersetzung mit der Psychologie C. G. Jungs*, ed. Ernst Michel and Arie Sborowitz with a preface by Martin Buber (Stuttgart: Ernst Klett Verlag, 1952).

soul. A soul is never sick alone, but always a between-ness also, a situation between it and another existing being. The psychotherapist who has passed through the crisis may now dare to touch on this.

This way of frightened pause, of unfrightened reflection, of personal involvement, of rejection of security, of unreserved stepping into relationship, of the bursting of psychologism, this way of vision and of risk is that which Hans Trüb trod. . . . Surely there will not be wanting men like him—awake and daring, hazarding the economics of the vocation, not sparing and not withholding themselves—men who will find his path and extend it further.[21]

This essay offers evidence that the men whom Buber called for do exist. One of the most interesting of these is the noted American psychologist, Carl R. Rogers. In a discussion of Ludwig Binswanger's "Case of Ellen West" which he entitles "The Loneliness of Contemporary Man," [22] Rogers points to Buber's "healing through meeting" as the center of therapy. The greatest weakness of Ellen West's treatment, in Rogers's opinion, was that no one involved in it seems to have related to her as a *person,* a person "whose inner experiencing is a precious resource to be drawn upon and trusted." She was dealt with as an object, helped to *see* her feelings but not to *experience* them. She herself recognized that the doctor could give her discernment but not healing. She uttered a desperate cry for a relationship between two persons, but no one heard her. "She never experienced what Buber has called 'healing through meeting.' There was no one who could meet her, accept her, as she was." Rogers draws from the case of Ellen

21. Martin Buber, *A Believing Humanism*, pp. 142–43.
22. *The Worlds of Existentialism*, pp. 484–85. For "The Case of Ellen West" itself, see Rollo May, Ernest Angel, Henri F. Ellenberger, eds., *Existence. A New Dimension in Psychiatry and Psychology* (New York: Basic Books, 1958), pp. 237–364.

West the lesson that in every respect in which the therapist makes an object of the person—"whether by diagnosing him, analyzing him, or perceiving him impersonally in a case history"—he stands in the way of his therapeutic goal. The therapist is deeply helpful only when he relates as a person, risks himself as a person in the relationship, experiences the other as a person in his own right. "Only then is there a meeting of a depth which dissolves the pain of aloneness in both client and therapist." [23]

In his book *On Becoming a Person*,[24] Rogers tells how he changed his approach to therapy from the intellectual question of how he could treat the patient to the recognition that changes come about through *experience* in a *relationship*. He found that the more genuine he was in a relationship, the more aware he was of his own feelings, the more willing he was to express his own feelings and attitudes, the more he gave the relationship a *reality* which the person could use for his own personal growth. He also found that the more he could respect and like the patient, showing a warm regard for him as a person of unconditional self-worth and accepting each fluctuating aspect of the other, the more he was creating a relationship which the individual could use. This acceptance necessarily includes a continuing desire to understand the other's feelings and thoughts, which leaves him really free to explore all the hidden nooks and frightening crannies of his inner and often buried experience. This also includes a complete freedom from any type of moral or diagnostic evaluation.

Rogers's "deep empathic understanding," which enables him to see his client's private world through his eyes, is close to Buber's "experiencing the other side," or "inclusion." Rogers states that "when I hold in myself the kind of attitudes I have

23. Ibid., pp. 484–85.

24. Carl R. Rogers, *On Becoming A Person. A Therapist's View of Psychotherapy* (Boston: Houghton Mifflin, 1961).

described, and when the other person can to some degree experience these attitudes, then I believe that change and constructive personal development will *invariably* occur." [25] This faith in the latent potentialities that will become actual "in a suitable psychological climate," seems to expect of "healing through meeting" an effectiveness which goes beyond the concrete situation with its often tragic limitations. If the parent creates such a psychological climate, "the child will become more self-directing, socialized, and mature," [26] says Rogers. Through relationship, the other individual will experience and understand the repressed aspects of himself, will become better integrated and more effective in functioning, closer to the person he would like to be, "more of a person, more unique and more self-expressive," and he "will be able to cope with the problems of life more adequately and more comfortably." [27]

In this connection Rogers uses Buber's phrase "confirming the other," that is, accepting the person not as something fixed and finished but as a process of becoming. Through this acceptance, says Rogers, "I am doing what I can to confirm or make real his potentialities." If, on the contrary, writes Rogers, one sees the relationship as merely an opportunity to reinforce certain types of words or opinions in the other, as Verplanck, Lindsley, and B. F. Skinner do in their therapy of operant conditioning, then one confirms him as a basically mechanical, manipulable object, and he tends to act in ways that support this hypothesis. Only the relationship which "reinforces" *all* that he is, "the person that he is with all his existent potentialities," Rogers concludes, is one that, to use Buber's term, *confirms* him "as a living person, capable of creative inner development." [28]

25. Ibid., chap. 2, p. 35.
26. Ibid., p. 37.
27. Ibid., p. 38.
28. Ibid., chap. 3, pp. 55–56.

Rogers's great affinity to Buber's "healing through meet-ing" [29] makes all the more significant those issues that arose between Rogers and Buber in their 1957 dialogue.[30] One of these was that of man's nature—can one trust his potentialities to be "good" and socially constructive providing he is accepted by the therapist and learns to accept himself, as Rogers holds? Or is man polar, as Buber contends, having potentialities that need direction and temptations to inauthenticity against which both he and the therapist must struggle? This issue is closely related to others that arose in this dialogue. One of these was Rogers's insistence on complete mutuality between himself and his client in contrast to Buber's insistence on the normative limitation in the therapeutic relationship, which adds to mutual contact and mutual trust the essentially nonmutual fact of the therapist's experiencing the patient's side of the relationship.

The patient can neither experience the therapist's side of the relationship nor see him as he really is, disentangled from the patient's own needs. Rogers *wants* his client to be on the same plane with him, but Buber says that there is also the *situation*, sometimes tragic, which Rogers cannot change. Rogers insists that, however unequally the relationship may be seen in the world of I-It, in the I-Thou meeting between therapist and client, he looks upon the client as having equal authority, equal validity in the way he sees life. He goes so far as to say that there is the same kind of meeting whether the person met is normal, a schizophrenic, or a paranoid. "The moments in which people *do* change, are the moments in

29. I have demonstrated this at great length and on the basis of Rogers's earlier book, *Client-Centered Therapy, Its Current Practice, Implications and Theory* (Boston: Houghton Mifflin Co., 1951), in my book, *Martin Buber: The Life of Dialogue* (New York: Harper Torchbooks, 1960), pp. 191–94.

30. Buber, *The Knowledge of Man*, appendix: "Dialogue between Martin Buber and Carl R. Rogers," moderated by Maurice Friedman.

which perhaps the relationship is experienced the same on both sides." [31] Buber's response is that Rogers, in saying this, is ignoring the limits that lead a schizophrenic to shut himself off from others and that shut a paranoid off without his willing it.

In my own role as moderator of this dialogue between Buber and Rogers, I suggested that the real difference was that Buber was stressing the client's inability to experience Rogers's side of the relationship, whereas Rogers was stressing the meeting, the change that takes place in the meeting, and his own *feeling* that the client is an equal person whom he respects. Rogers replied that in the most real moments of therapy the intention to help is only a substratum. Although he would not say that the relationship is reciprocal in the sense that the client wants to understand him and help him, he does assert that when real change takes place it is reciprocal in the sense that the therapist sees this individual as he *is* in that moment, and the client really senses his understanding and acceptance of him. To this Buber replied that Rogers gives the client something in order to make him equal for that moment, but that this is a situation of minutes, not of an hour, and these minutes are made possible by Rogers who, "out of a certain fullness," gives the client what he wants in order to be *able* to be, just for this moment, on the same plane with him.

A second issue that arose was whether what Rogers means by *accepting* the person is the same as what Buber means by *confirming* the person. Rogers, as we have seen, does equate these two. True acceptance, he holds, means acceptance of this person's potentialities as well as what he is at the moment. If we were not able to recognize his potentiality, Rogers says, it is a real question whether we could accept him. If I am accepted exactly as I am, he adds, I cannot help but change. When there is no longer any need for defensive barriers, the

31. Ibid., p. 175.

forward-moving processes of life take over. It is precisely this assumption—that the processes of life will always be forward-moving—which Buber questions, and this leads him to a distinction between affirmation and confirmation that Rogers does not make:

> Every true existential relationship between two persons begins with acceptance. . . . I take you just as you are . . . in this moment, in this actuality. . . . Confirming means . . . accepting the whole potentiality of the other and even making a decisive difference in his potentiality. . . . I can recognize in him, know in him, more or less, the person he has been . . . *created* to become. . . . And now I not only accept the other as he is, but I confirm him, in myself and then in him, in relation to this potentiality that . . . can now be developed, . . . can evolve, . . . can answer the reality of life. . . . "I accept you as you are." . . . does *not* mean "I don't want you to change," but . . . "I discover in you just by my accepting love . . . what you are meant to become." [32]

Buber goes on to say that in working with a problematic man he must sometimes help him against himself, for because of this problematic, life has become baseless for him.

> What he wants is a being not only whom he can trust as a man trusts another, but a being that gives him now the certitude that "there *is* a soil, there *is* an existence. The world is not condemned to deprivation, degeneration, destruction. The world *can* be redeemed. *I* can be redeemed because there is this trust." And if this is reached, now I can help this man even in his struggle against himself. And this I can only do if I distinguish between accepting and confirming. [33]

32. Ibid., pp. 181–82.
33. Ibid., p. 183.

The German psychiatrist Viktor von Weizsäcker[34] places healing through meeting at the center of his "medical anthropology," which begins with the recognition of the difference between the objective understanding of some*thing* and the "transjective" understanding of some*one*. The doctor can only understand the patient if he begins with questions addressed to a person rather than with objective knowledge about an object. Only through the real contact of doctor and patient does objective science have a part in the history of the latter's illness. If this contact is lacking, all information about functions, drives, properties, and capacities is falsified. This comradeship of doctor and patient takes place not despite technique and rational thought but through and with them. The smooth functioning of the objective practitioner lasts just as long as there is a self-understood relation between doctor and patient, unnoticed because unthreatened. But if this de facto assent to the relationship falls away, then the objectivity is doubtful and no longer of use.

Von Weizsäcker expands this relationship of doctor and patient into an all-embracing distinction between objective therapy and "inclusive," or "comprehensive" therapy, using the latter word in Buber's sense of *Umfassung*, or experiencing the other side of the relationship. The most important characteristic of an inclusive therapy, in von Weizsäcker's opinion, is that the doctor allows himself to be changed by the patient, that he allows all the impulses that proceed from the person of the patient to affect him, that he is receptive not only with the objective sense of sight but also with hearing, which brings the I and Thou together. Only through this ever-new involvement of his personality can the doctor bring his capacities to full realization in his relation with his patient.

Only through this conscious dominion of a *relationship* over the psychic process, in this long and from-case-to-case-

34. "Doctor and Patient" (selections) in *The Worlds of Existentialism*, pp. 405–07.

ever-newly-offered chain of sacrifices and new involve-
ments of the personality, can the doctor be educated in
that which enables him to encompass the resistances and
to set the projected goal beyond the circumscribed area of
objective therapy.[35]

It helps in this process if the doctor recognizes that even the
needs that cut the patient off, physical or psychic, are facts of
the relationship between man and man, variants which call
that relationship forth to another level. On the other hand,
that objective approach to therapy which leads the judging
mind to disengage itself from the moment of the experiencing
contact, rests on a false image of man: "He is then thought of
as a being of size, surface, area, weight, function, desire,
consciousness, characteristics and capabilities of all sorts," [36]
all of which are false judgments, false images. Von Weizsäcker
applies this dialogical approach even to psychotics. What
makes us mistrustful of many psychotics, he writes, is that their
self-deification and self-degradation lack all moderation. The
cause of this overvaluation of the self is the isolation of the
psychotic, the fact that he has no Thou for his I. The result of
the absence of a Thou is an inner double. This illusion of the
double is unavoidable after a man has lost his connection with
a Thou, writes von Weizsäcker, for the state of aloneness that
he has reached then is unbearable. "The cleavage of the I
represents—for a moment—the relationship of the I to the
Thou which has become unattainable." [37]

The reciprocity of relationships is without doubt the least
explored part of medical anthropology until now, says von
Weizsäcker. When one arrives at the very ground of events,
explanations cease and things are as they are. But "the
relationship of man to man plays a powerful role, and in this

35. Ibid., p. 408
36. Ibid., p. 407.
37. Ibid., Viktor von Weizsäcker, "Cases and Problems" (selections), p. 409.

relationship first arises much of that which one calls ability, character, disposition and heredity." Pathology after Freud must be not only individual but also social, he concludes.[38]

One of the most significant contributions to our understanding of healing through meeting is the work of Leslie H. Farber, chairman of the Association for Existential Psychology and Psychiatry. Under the influence of Buber, as well as of Kierkegaard and his former mentor Harry Stack Sullivan, Farber has developed an original theory of "will and willfulness" as the center of psychiatric diagnosis and healing. Farber's approach to psychotherapy is essentially dialogical. At the same time, he has gone further than anyone in recognizing the terribly tragic limitations of healing through meeting to which Buber points in his dialogue with Rogers.

In his essay on "Martin Buber and Psychoanalysis," [39] Farber affirms that without meeting no successful treatment is possible. The "compulsive," "schizoid" or "hysterical" traits that therapist and patient have in conmon only indicate that both have an incapacity in common that hinders the meeting. Many of the disturbances that are seen as arising from "transference" are more correctly described as the striving for, or retreating from, the hope for a reciprocal relationship. Usually what we mean by "transference" is the very opposite of meeting, with its warmth, contact, and spontaneity. What is important, however, is to combine reciprocity or trust with truthfulness and proportion. These two can combine into a unique immediacy: meeting becomes truth.

At the same time, Farber emphasizes that Buber's philosophy is based as much upon the necessary structures and categories of the world of It as the bringing of those structures and categories into the meeting with the Thou.

> The mistake is often made, especially with the schizophrenic, of overvaluing his lonely gropings toward the

---

38. Ibid., p. 410.

39. Leslie H. Farber, *The Ways of the Will. Essays Toward A Psychology and Psychopathology of Will* (New York: Basic Books, 1966), chap. 7.

Thou and of underestimating his actual incompetence in the world of *It*, so that he becomes a tragic saint or poet of the *Thou*, martyred by the world of *It*.

Once it is realized, however, that the *Thou* relation depends upon the world of *It* for its conceptual forms or meanings, then psychosis can be seen as not only a failure of the *Thou*—of so-called personal relations. It is an equal failure of knowledge, judgment, and experience in the world of *It*. Whatever class the disorder falls into— whether it is marked by a recoil from relations, as in schizophrenia, or by a grasping at relation, as in hysteria or mania—underlying its manifestations one can always find much ineptitude with people, much early failure to acquire the elementary tools of knowledge. . . . Without sufficient knowledge, memory, or judgment, every *Thou* invoked is apt to be a perilously shy and fleeting one. It recedes very quickly into its impoverished world of *It*, where there is little promise of return. And with each loss of the *Thou*, the schizophrenic is in special danger of retreating more permanently or deeply toward his far pole of alienation: into that *loneliness* of which both Sullivan and Fromm-Reichmann have written.[40]

Farber describes this loneliness as a hopeless longing for the Thou, a despair which afflicts everyone at times "and overwhelms the more desperate ones we call psychotic." In this sense, the chatter by which we detain even an unwelcome guest when he is parting is no less a confession of the total failure of the wedding of minds than that even madder chattering by which the "manic" patient detains all humanity as his parting guest. "We strive wildly on the doorstep for one departing *Thou*." For the schizophrenic, this often means that the longing for the Thou is accompanied by a fear of his

40. Ibid., pp. 148–49.

loneliness being momentarily entered by a Thou and then
leaving him all the more desolate and empty-handed when he
returns to the vacant world of It. Unable to endure this
possibility, he "exiles himself from both earth and heaven,
and, with a surprising dignity, takes up his residence in
limbo." [41] The sickness arising from lack of dialogue thus
makes itself worse by striving in desperate or inadequate ways
for the Thou, or by fearing the loneliness that will follow the
fleeting appearance of the Thou.

It is within this context that Farber develops his contrast
between genuine will and arbitrary willfulness, the former an
expression of real dialogue, the latter a hysterical product of
the absence of dialogue. In contrast to Freud, who sees hysteria
as a product of repression which can be cured by bringing the
repressed material to consciousness, Farber defines hysteria as
a disorder of the will that expresses itself in *willfulness*. "In
willfulness the life of the will becomes distended, overweening,
and obtrusive at the same time that its movements become
increasingly separate, sovereign, and distinct from other
aspects of spirit." [42] This leads to that very failure of discretion
and judgment, as well as imagination and humor, which
Farber points to as the inadequacy of the schizophrenic in the
world of It as well as in the relationship with the Thou.

The origin of willfulness Farber sees as the desperate need
for wholeness. The proper setting of wholeness is dialogue.
When this setting eludes us, "we turn wildly to will, ready to
grasp at any illusion of wholeness (however mindless or
grotesque) the will conjures up for our reassurance." [43] This is
a vicious circle, for the more dependent a person becomes on
the illusion of wholeness, the less he is able to experience true
wholeness in dialogue. "At the point where he is no longer

41. Ibid., pp. 149–50.
42. Ibid., chap. 5, "Will and Willfulness in Hysteria," p. 103.
43. Ibid., p. 111.

capable of dialogue he can be said to be *addicted* to his will." [44]
Willfulness, then, is nothing other than the attempt of will to
make up for the absence of dialogue by handling both sides of
the no longer mutual situation. No longer in encounter with
another self, he fills the emptiness with his own self, and even
that self is only a partial one, its wholeness having disappeared
with the disappearance of meeting. "This feverish figure,
endlessly assaulting the company, seeking to wrench the
moment to some pretense of dialogue, is the image of the
eternal stranger: that condition of man in which he is forever
separated from his fellows, unknown and unaddressed—it is
the figure of man's separated will posing as his total self." [45]

In "Will and Anxiety" Farber defines anxiety, in conscious
contrast to his teacher Harry Stack Sullivan, as a product of
the separated, or isolated, will.

> By whatever name it is called, *anxiety is that range of distress
> which attends willing what cannot be willed.* In other words,
> anxiety can be located in the ever-widening split between
> the will and the impossible object of the will. As the split
> widens, the bondage between the will and its object
> grows, so that one is compelled to pursue what seems to
> wither or altogether vanish in the face of such pursuit.[46]

The more stubbornly the will pursues its intractable goal, the
more it becomes separate from those faculties of intellect and
imagination which might objectify, divert, or dispel its bondage. The failure of meaning that characterizes anxiety stems
from the withering of the will's goal in the face of the will's
demands. In contrast to the customary distinction between
fear as specific and anxiety as diffuse, Farber suggests that fear
merges into anxiety when willing what cannot be willed takes

44. Ibid.
45. Ibid., p. 117.
46. Ibid., chap. 2, p. 42.

over. At this point the will itself comes to be experienced as impotent thrust, resulting in the helplessness and uncertainty which characterize anxiety.

Rather than call this the Age of Anxiety, Farber calls it the Age of the Disordered Will. We are enslaved, he says, by myriad varieties of willing what cannot be willed: to sleep, to read fast, to have simultaneous orgasm, to be creative and spontaneous, to enjoy old age. Above all, it is the *will to will* that makes anxiety so prominent in our time and explains the increasing dependence on drugs in all levels of our society. More important than their function in relieving anxiety is the illusion drugs offer of healing the split between the will and its refractory object. This illusion offers, briefly and subjectively, the appearance of a responsible and vigorous will. This is the reason, in Farber's opinion, why the addictive possibilities of our age are so enormous.

We experience "a mounting hunger for a sovereign and irreducible will, so wedded to our reason, our emotions, our imagination, our intentions, our bodies, that only after a given enterprise has come to an end can we retrospectively infer that will was present at all." [47] This is the will of the whole being rather than of isolated willfulness, of freedom rather than bondage, of dialogue rather than monologue. Farber suggests that both the disordered will and the hunger for the whole will of dialogue may be understood in terms of our position on the far side of "the death of God." For Dostoievski's Kirilov in *The Possessed*, it was possible to assert: "To recognize that there is no God and not to recognize at the same instant that one is God oneself is an absurdity, else one would certainly kill oneself." Standing on the other side of the divide, the loss has penetrated and shaped our life in subtle, pedestrian ways that make the position of Dostoievski's man-god, the "Modern Promethean," an outworn vestige of romanticism.[48] Man is not

47. Ibid., p. 48.
48. For my discussion of Kirilov as a modern Promethean, see Maurice Friedman,

even for Farber what he is for Sartre in *Being and Nothingness*, "a useless passion." After the death of God, we do not try to become God ourselves but settle instead for the isolated, disordered will of willfulness.

> With the disappearance of the divine Will from our lives, we have come to hunger not for *His Will*—neither in the sense of living *in* His Will nor *usurping* His Will for ourselves—but rather for our *own* sovereign will, which is our modern way, this side the omnipotence of suicide or madness. And all exhortations notwithstanding, this will we cannot will.[49]

One way out of the impasse of the disordered will may be despair, Farber suggests, in "Schizophrenia and the Mad Psychotherapist." Despair may provide "the very conditions of seriousness and urgency which bring a man to ask those wholly authentic—we might call them tragic—questions about his own life and the meaning and measure of his particular humanness." [50] When despair is repudiated, these questions may mark the turning to the inauthentic. This applies to the therapist, too, who *wills* relation. True relationship cannot be willed; it depends on honesty, imagination, tact, humor. "By contrast, the willful encounter . . . will have a special binge-like excitement, even though its center is hollow. Its intensity is of the moment." This drama of wills that passes for relation finally turns the therapist into "an apostle of relation who can no longer abide relation." As the therapist continues to will what cannot be willed, his human qualities progressively atrophy in favor of "those public,

---

Problematic Rebel: Melville, Dostoievsky, Kafka, Camus, 2d ed., enlarged and radically reorganized (Chicago: The University of Chicago Press and Phoenix Books [paperback], 1970), pp. 182–89.

49. Farber, *The Ways of the Will*, chap. 2, "Will and Anxiety," p. 50.

50. Ibid., chap. 9, p. 196.

self-assertive gestures which are inauthentic to the person he might have become." [51]

Farber's implicit conclusion is that if patient and therapist alike are to have any hope of reaching real dialogue, they must be willing to face the despair which occupies so central a place even in the attempt at healing through meeting. This despair must be distinguished from that pseudo-despair which leads to "the life of suicide." The very strategies of despair involved in the contemplation of suicide reveal a link to the life-outside-despair that despair is unable to sever. "Despair would not be so anguished a condition as it is were it as wholly and hopelessly estranged as it believes itself to be." [52] Even if the life of suicide issues in actual suicide, this does not mean that the despair was as total as the despairer thinks. The man who commits suicide imagines he has made a bargain with death. Through death he will be able to find the last and grandest expression of willfulness—"the dramatic representation of some uniqueness, some singularity of self with which life has seemingly so far failed to provide him, and of which his natural—un-self-engineered—death threatens to rob him." This ultimate perversion of dialogue is "a dream of the will—a despairing attempt to affirm the self in a form in which the self has never been and can never be." [53]

One of the most remarkable conclusions that Farber draws is that the genuineness of despair not only may lead the therapist to face the true situation in regard to his "dialogue" with his schizophrenic patient, but may even lead the patient to moments of pity for the therapist, through which, for those moments at least, the patient transcends his schizophrenia and enters into dialogue. Thus, though the therapist may not demand that the patient see the relationship from his point of

51. Ibid., pp. 207–08.
52. Ibid., chap. 4, "Despair and the Life of Suicide," p. 96.
53. Ibid., pp. 97–98.

view, it is possible with a schizophrenic that he may do so, and
that precisely here will lie the "healing through meeting" that
takes place. Making use of Buber's concepts of presentness and
confirmation, Farber suggests that only that therapist who is
capable of arousing pity by becoming "present" for his patient
will be able to help the patient. When the patient is able to
make the therapist present, to "imagine the real" in relation to
him, he becomes capable of pity for his friend's distress. "In
response to the therapist's despair . . . the patient will often
try to confirm the therapist's image of himself as therapist.
And insofar as the therapist is sincerely dedicated to his work
. . . this will also have the effect of confirming him as a fellow
human being." [54] Thus, in a way that goes beyond any
envisaged by Buber himself, Farber uses Buber's theory of
confirmation to distinguish between the dialogue between
therapist and patient and the more fully mutual dialogue of
friendship and love.

In moving into the realm of healing through meeting, we
must face the radical question of whether true healing, in the
first instance, is not *psycho*therapy but rather family, social,
economic, and political therapy. The readjustment and integration of the intrapsychic sphere is the *byproduct,* but the locus
of true healing is the interhúman, the interpersonal, the
communal, the social, the cultural, and even the political. To
embark seriously on healing through meeting is to leave the
safe shores of the intrapsychic as *the* touchstone of reality and
to venture onto the high seas in which healing is no longer
seen as something taking place *in* the patient. Although one
hopes that the client becomes wholer in the process, and
although the therapist has a special role as initiator, facilitator, confidant, big brother, and representative of the dialogical
demand of the world, the healing itself takes place in that

54. Ibid., chap. 8, "The Therapeutic Despair," p. 171.

sphere which Buber calls the "between." Nor can this healing
be limited to the client alone, or even to the relationship
between therapist and client. To be real healing, it must
eventually burst the bounds of *psycho*therapy and enter in all
seriousness into the interhuman, the family, the group, the
community, and even the relations between communities and
nations. In his address to the Jungian Psychological Club of
Zurich in 1923, on "The Psychologizing of the World," Buber
explicitly pointed to the problematic limits of the province of
psychotherapy and the need for healing to transcend that
sphere:

> The sicknesses of the soul are sicknesses of relationship.
> They can only be treated completely if I transcend the
> realm of the patient and add to it the world as well. If the
> doctor possessed superhuman power, he would have to try
> to heal the relationship itself, to heal in the "between."
> The doctor must know that really he ought to do that and
> that only his boundedness limits him to the one side.[55]

Today many family therapists, such as Ronald Laing and
Lyman Wynne, recognize the truth of what Buber said and go
beyond the advocacy of only one side of the relationship. The
most decisive breakthrough to healing through meeting
beyond the intrapsychic has been the work of Ivan Boszormenyi-Nagy, Director of the Family Psychiatry Division of the
Eastern Pennsylvania Psychiatric Institute in Philadelphia.
Hans Trüb, Leslie Farber, Ronald Laing, and Sidney Jourard
have already made explicit use of Buber's understanding of
confirmation and of the primacy of meeting, or dialogue, in
their approach to therapy.

Only Nagy, to my knowledge, has built his therapy on the
further reaches of Buber's philosophical anthropology—his
understanding of the "essential We," the common world built
by the common "speech-with-meaning" and the existential

55. Buber, *A Believing Humanism*, p. 150.

guilt that arises from the injury to this common world.[56] The "common cosmos" of the We is no universal ideal metaphysical order but the world that we actually build among ourselves through our common "logos" of speech-with-meaning. Guilt, therefore—real existential guilt—has to do with the injuring of this order of being. In contrast to the neurotic guilt that is repressed into the unconscious, the event which produces existential guilt remains conscious, even though it is not remembered as guilt. Also in contrast to neurotic guilt, which often is an impersonal breaking of social taboos, existential guilt is personal guilt that we take upon ourselves as persons. Yet it is not merely in us. It is, most important of all, a real injury to the order of being, the foundations of which we recognize as those of our own existence and of those with whom we live in community.

In *Invisible Loyalties*,[57] the decisive formulation of his relational theory and family therapy, Nagy declares the intrapsychic realm meaningless if it is taken out of the context of the I-Thou relationship. If this is so, the client cannot solve his problems with his family, as so many traditionally oriented psychoanalysts recommend, just by moving away from home and becoming independent or by bringing to consciousness his feelings of hatred for his parents. A mass escape from filial obligations through fear of responsibility can infuse all human relationships with unbearable chaos, Nagy says. The individual can become paralyzed by amorphous, undefinable existential guilt. By the same token, "the true measure of human emotion is not the intensity of its affective or physiological

56. See Buber, *The Knowledge of Man*, chap. 1, "Introductory Essay" by Maurice Friedman; chap. 4, "What Is Common to All"; and chap. 6, "Guilt and Guilt Feelings."

57. Ivan Boszormenyi-Nagy and Geraldine M. Spark, *Invisible Loyalties. Reciprocity in Intergenerational Family Therapy* (New York: Harper & Row, Medical Division, 1973). I refer in this essay only to Ivan B.-Nagy because it is he who authored the main theoretical chapters.

concomitant, but the relevance of its interpersonal context." [58]
Nagy follows Buber in distinguishing between relationships
which are merely functions of individual becoming, normalcy,
adaptation, and perspective, and relationships which are
ontological in the sense that they have a reality, meaning, and
value in themselves. This leads Nagy to forceful and repeated
emphasis on Buber's distinction between *intrapsychic guilt feelings*
and *interhuman existential guilt.*

> The therapist who wants to liberate the patient from his
> concern for or guilt-laden loyalty to members of his
> family may succeed in removing certain manifestations of
> psychological guilt, but may at the same time increase the
> patient's existential guilt. Buber distinguished between
> guilt feelings and existential guilt. The latter obviously
> goes beyond psychology: It has to do with objective harm
> to the order and justice of the human world. If I really
> betrayed a friend or if my mother really feels that I
> damaged her through my existence, the reality of a
> disturbed order of the human world remains, whether I
> can get rid of certain guilt feelings or not. Such guilt
> becomes part of a systemic ledger of merits and can only
> be affected by action and existential rearrangement, if at
> all.[59]

Nagy sees the "invisible loyalties"—the commitment and
devotion that are important determinants in family relationships—as making for a deeper binding than the genuine
I-Thou dialogue that is possible between those who are not
related. My son is "a unique counterpart of my existential
realm," whose meaning for me cannot be embodied by anyone
else, for it is part of a multigenerational relationship system
which he and I share. Nor can talking *about* family relation-

58. Ibid., p. 13.
59. Ibid., p. 184.

ships in group therapy or encounter groups take the place of actual family therapy, for it lacks "the pressure of relevance, which gives relational therapy its greatest leverage." [60]

This does not mean that the therapist does not play a part in the healing through meeting that takes place in family therapy. The family therapist must be open and expose himself, and he must let this affect his relationship to his own family. "It is our conviction that growth in our personal life is not only inseparable from growth in our professional experience, but that it is our greatest technical tool." [61] At the same time "transference" in the family therapy system has a very different meaning from what it has in individual therapy. Freud could speak of the patient's self-deception concerning the nature of the patient/doctor relationship as a cognitive error, a distortion in perception and thinking. Family system therapists, in contrast, are more interested in the existential implications of transference. Transferred attitudes and expectations carry the continuity of past, unresolved obligations and expectations of family systems, and signify factual events. This means that positive transference to the therapist is not always possible or desirable since it can amount to intrinsic disloyalty to the rejected parent.

Nagy's goals of family therapy are best understood in terms of Buber's anthropology of *distancing* and *relating* as the two ontological movements fundamental to human existence. To Nagy, therapy can never stop with getting out the buried hostility toward the parents; for that would inevitably lead to a division of loyalties, a rejection of the therapist, or a building up of guilt. "In our clinical experience, no one ends up a winner through a conclusion which predicates a hopelessly incorrigible resentment and contempt towards one's parent."

While conscious confrontation with one's hateful feelings amounts to progress, it does not represent a therapeutic

60. Ibid., p. 93.
61. Ibid., p. 13.

endpoint. Unless the person can struggle with his negative feelings and resolve them by acts based on positive, helpful attitudes towards his parent, he cannot really free himself of the intrinsic loyalty problem and has to "live" the conflict, even after the parent's death, through pathological defensive patterns.[62]

Intergenerational loyalty means that frequently the outcome is the rejection and scapegoating of the therapist in order to escape from the annihilating effect of victory over one's parents. "The cost of such victory would be guilt, shame, and a paradoxically binding loyalty, disowned, denied, yet paralyzingly adhered to at the same time." [63]

The positive goal of therapy is a dialectic between individuation and family loyalty, for the former cannot be achieved at the cost of simply severing family ties. Every step leading toward the child's true emancipation "tends to touch on the emotionally charged issue of every member's denied but wished-for everlasting symbiotic togetherness with the family of origin." [64] The pathological expression of the failure to achieve this balance is what Murray Bowen calls the "undifferentiated ego mass," or the "polarized fusion of roles," where instead of a genuinely antithetical dialogue between unique persons, people are symbiotically related through roles. "The individual can be liberated to engage in full, wholly personal relationships only to the extent that he has become capable of responding to parental devotion with concern." [65] Thus, what is central to Buber in *I and Thou*—learning to meet others and hold one's ground when one meets them—is central to Nagy's family therapy. Individual autonomy is not viewed mainly within the confines of ego strength and intrapsychic

62. Ibid., p. 20.
63. Ibid.
64. Ibid., p. 21.
65. Ibid., p. 105.

resourcefulness and effective adaptation, as in individual
therapy, but is in a dynamically antithetic relationship with
loyalty to the family of origin.

One of Nagy's most important concepts, correspondingly, is
that of "parentification," in which the parent has given the
burden of parenting to the child, perhaps because of inadequate parenting by his own parents of origin. The rebellion of
the so-called delinquent child may actually be, from this
viewpoint, an attempt to bring the feuding parents together,
and the identified patient in the family, the "schizophrenic,"
may really be the scapegoat who bears the problems of the
family. There may even arise a basic trust among siblings who
share in common the parentification thrust upon them by
their parents. The loss of a meaningful relationship, either
through rejection of the child by the parents or through the
child's becoming autonomous and moving away from the
parents, "always implies the ontic disconfirmation of one's
person," [66] says Nagy. Thus the threat of separation becomes
one of the most important dynamics that must be recognized
in Nagy's system of family therapy:

> Man's greatest satisfaction is connected with entering into
> a relationship, and his greatest pain with unrelatedness or
> the threat of losing an important relationship. As the
> chance of raising a family is the most universal source of
> anticipated happiness, the prospect of losing one's child,
> even through the child's growth and maturation, can lead
> to the most penetrating grief.[67]

In contrast to those family therapists who hold that the
therapist must not judge, Nagy espouses a "multidirectional
partiality" in which the therapist will be partial at one time to
one member of the family and at another time to another. The

66. Ibid., p. 154.
67. Ibid., p. 153.

family therapist must be strong enough to be included in the
family system as present for each and every member, yet
remain outside in the role of facilitator for emotional change
and growth. He must have that "inclusion" of which Buber
speaks, by which the therapist "imagines the real"—that is,
experiences the patient's side of the relationship without losing
his own. But there is also a demand that he places on the
members of the family.

> The contract means that the therapist has to offer and
> actually make himself available as willing to help all
> members, whether they come to therapy sessions or not.
> In turn, he has to extract commitment for participation
> from all members of the family. He wants all those
> present to expose their opinions, needs, and wishes for
> help, and he tries to make sure that the messages of even
> the smallest child are being heard and responded to.[68]

The culmination of Nagy's family therapy is reciprocal
justicing that rebalances the "merit ledger" between the
generations. This can be done only through listening to each
member's subjective construction of his accountability to the
rest of the family. Nagy's touchstone of reality is not functional
efficiency but the intrinsic balances between hidden loyalty
ties and exploitations. This leads, in turn, to what I have
called the "dialogue of touchstones," in which each person's
point of view is confirmed precisely through coming into
dialogue with the opposing views of others. The goal of Nagy's
family therapy is not the community of affinity, or like-
mindedness, but what I call the "community of otherness." [69]
In marriage, it is not just two individuals who join but two

68. Ibid., p. 16.
69. See Maurice Friedman, *Touchstones of Reality. Existential Trust and the Community of Peace* (New York: Dutton Books [paperback], 1974); and Maurice Friedman, *The Hidden Human Image* (New York: Delacorte Press and Delta Books [paperback], 1974), chap. 19, "The Community of Otherness and the Covenant of Peace."

quite different family systems of merit. If one does not intuitively perceive this, one marries the other only in fantasy, as the wishfully improved re-creation of one's own family of origin. Each mate may then struggle to coerce the other to be accountable for those of his or her felt injustices and accrued merit which come from his or her family of origin. By improving their reciprocal loyalty exchange with their families of origin, Nagy's family therapy helps the married couple relate to each other and to their children.

Thus, confirmation in the dialogue of touchstones leading to the community of otherness is both the way and the goal of Nagy's family therapy. "Personal exploitation is measurable only on a subjective scale which has been built into the person's sense of the meaning of his entire existence." [70] Being confirmed is not a matter of the *quantity* of the world's goods that one gets, but of "a reality-based or action dialogue, which is more than the sum total of two persons' subjective experiences." [71] The concept of reality-testing in Freudian psychology is a comparatively monological one, in which the patient is either reality-bound or subject to distortion. This means, as Ronald Laing has pointed out, that the psychiatrist determines what is "normal" and invalidates the experience of the patient. And it means, as Nagy has stressed, that "the psychotherapist, together with his patient, develop what is 'normal' and implicitly invalidate the experience and needs of all partners to the patient's close relationships." [72]

Buber's and Nagy's concept of "the just order of the human world," in contrast, is a dialogical one. However pathological it may be, the unique experience of each of the persons in the family is itself of value: it enters into the balance of merit and into the dialogical reality-testing—the "dialogue of touch-

70. *Invisible Loyalties*, p. 81.
71. Ibid., p. 82.
72. Letter from Nagy to Maurice Friedman, June 21, 1974.

stones." The scapegoater in the family can be looked upon as needing help and the scapegoat as a potential helper; for the former is taking an ever-heavier load of guilt on himself and the latter is accumulating merit through being loaded on by others. Justice is, for Nagy, "a personal principle of equity of mutual give and take which guides the individual member of a social group in facing the ultimate consequences of his relationships with others." [73] The climate of trust that characterizes a social entity is the sum total of the subjective evaluations of the justice of each member's relational experiences within what Nagy calls the "revolving slate" of the historically formed merit ledger.

> We believe that the "interhuman" realm of justice of the human world is the foundation of the prospects of trust among people. . . . Attempts at denying or escaping from such accounting constitute a major dynamic of every relationship system. While such escape may be necessary temporarily for the person's autonomous explorations, it must be uncovered and faced if the social system is to remain productive of healthy growth.[74]

Insight alone—the confrontation with the merit ledger—is only the preface to the task of actively balancing relationships. In *The Knowledge of Man*, Martin Buber sees the overcoming of existential guilt as taking place through the three stages of illuminating that guilt, persevering in that illumination, and repairing the injured order of being by reentering the dialogue with the world. In exact parallel, Nagy sees knowledge of the self and increased assertiveness as finding their place in the context of the accounts of fairness and justice in close relationships. No matter how vindictive a person may feel, the therapeutic goal must ultimately be focused on mutual

73. *Invisible Loyalties*, p. 61.
74. Ibid., p. 148.

clarification and reconstruction in order to provide the adult child and his parents with the opportunity to break the destructive, chainlike patterns of relationship which may have continued for several generations. The injustice of the parentification of children by their parents can only be redressed if one first goes back to the relationships of the parents to their own families of origin and does something about constructive repayment of indebtedness there. The family therapist must help the children give up their assumed adultlike roles.

In order to accomplish this, however, it is first necessary that the adults' unmet dependency needs and unresolved negative loyalty ties, based on unjust treatment and exploitation by their families of origin, be recognized and worked through—wherever possible with the families of origin themselves. In many cases even the terminal illness of the old parent offers the opportunity for repayment of obligations and subsequent emotional liberation of all three generations from guilt. "We believe that the major avenue toward interrupting the multigenerational chain of injustices goes via repairing relationships, and not through the dichotomy of either magnifying or denying the injury done to particular members." [75] One of the great opportunities of Nagy and Spark's three-generational approach lies in the possibility of rehabilitating the member's painful and shameful image of his parents through helping the member to understand the burdens laid on his parents by their own families of origin.

By opening up the door to rebalancing merits through action, the process of family therapy may reverse the accumulation and perpetuation of loaded, unsettled accounts which prejudice the chances of future generations. This applies even to the so-called paranoid.

> If a human being has been too deeply hurt and exploited
> to be able to absorb his wounds, he is entitled to a

75. Ibid., p. 95.

therapeutic recognition of the reality of his wounds and to a serious examination of the others' willingness to repair the damage. Only through such a "concession by the world" will he be prepared to reflect on the possible injustice of his own actions to others. . . . The badly hurt paranoid person should be given an extra chance, at least to the extent that the unfair balance of his justice is recognized. Whereas the reality of each member's early exploitation is anchored in the family's multigenerational ledger, each individual family member's sense of suffered injustice becomes his life-long programming for "emotional distortions," a psychological reality.[76]

Justice, like basic trust, characterizes the emotional climate and the existential ledger of a relationship system. Both concepts lie beyond the realm of individual psychology, and both lead to a reexamination and redefinition of the theories of projection, reality testing, fixation, displacement, transference, change, ego strength, and autonomy. From the standpoint of the relationship system, paranoia, for example, may be a perfectly rational state of mind. While it may be overreacting to a particular person, it still grows out of a real ethical imbalance of the past.

This redefinition of traditional psychological terms also leads Nagy to insight into the application of his dynamic of justice to the larger society as a whole. The "generation gap" is not one of communication but of justice, Nagy claims. "Retributory projection in all parent-like persons might be an important component of the hostility that exists between youth and the older generation in any culture." [77] Here, healing through meeting goes over in all explicitness to the community of otherness. "The greatest cultural task of our age," writes Nagy, "might be the investigation of the role of relational, not

76. Ibid., p. 91.
77. Ibid., p. 66.

merely economic justice, in contemporary society. And the greatest gap in our social science pertains to the denial of the psychological significance of retributive social dynamics." [78]

78. Ibid., p. 74.

10

On Death and Lying

Even the most humane studies of death are still permeated by
prejudices. Nineteen hundred years of Christian teaching have
left their mark on non-Christians, too. Consider two books
whose central motivation is altogether admirable: A. Alvarez,
The Savage God: A Study of Suicide (1971),[1] and Elisabeth
Kübler-Ross, *On Death and Dying* (1969).[2] Both books have won
wide attention, and Kübler-Ross continues to be a focal point
of discussion. Yet even authors of such caliber make unwarranted assumptions.

Alvarez has shown very fully—writing beautifully—how
suicide was at one time regarded without horror and loathing.
His chapter on "The Background" goes back far into the past,
while the chapters on "Suicide and Literature" quote writers
closer to us, like Montaigne, Shakespeare, John Donne, David
Hume, and many others, including some twentieth-century
writers. And yet we find Alvarez saying: "This is not to say
people commit suicide, as the Stoics did, coolly, deliberately,
as a rational choice between rational alternatives. The Ro-
mans may have disciplined themselves into accepting this
frigid logic, but those who have done so in modern history are,
in the last analysis, monsters" (pp. 120–21). The evidence that

1. London: Weidenfeld and Nicolson, 1971; New York: Random House, 1972.
2. New York: Macmillan, 1969. Citations refer to the paperback ed., New York:
Macmillan, 1970.

Alvarez himself presents so movingly does not in any way support this emotional outburst; and it is to his credit that he immediately proceeds to give an example that seems to contradict him: "In 1735 John Robeck, a Swedish philosopher living in Germany, completed a long Stoic defense of suicide . . . ; he then carefully put his principles into practice by giving away his property and drowning himself in the Weser." Surely, Robeck was no monster. But the case against Alvarez's claim does not depend on this one example. As already mentioned, he himself shows at length how Montaigne and Shakespeare, Donne and Hume, and many others, did not view suicide as he does.

There are at least two reasons for mentioning Alvarez. First, he cites a wealth of evidence to show how contemporary attitudes toward suicide are culturally conditioned. Secondly, he nevertheless shares some of the prejudices that he undermines.

Much the same is true of Kübler-Ross. Her cast of mind is more dogmatic than Alvarez's. On the opening pages of her book she makes some totally unsupported claims with an air of absolute certainty, insisting, for example, on the "*basic knowledge* that, in our unconscious, death is never possible in regard to ourselves" (p. 2, italics mine). This article of psychoanalytic faith she brings to her investigation and maintains *in spite* of the data she herself presents so movingly.

Her first chapter is called "On the Fear of Death," but nothing in that chapter supports her dogmatic claim that "the fear of death is a universal fear even if we think we have mastered it on many levels" (p. 5). This sweeping statement, thrown out at the start, is soon contradicted by her very first case history: "he was not afraid to die, but was afraid to live" (p. 20). Under the circumstances described by her, this seems an eminently rational and plausible attitude. Again, she explains very well how some students project their own feelings "onto the patients. The last has occasionally happened when a patient apparently faced death with calmness and equanimity while the student was highly upset by the encounter. The discussion then revealed that the student thought the patient was unrealistic or even faking, because it was inconceivable to him that anyone could face such a crisis with so much dignity" (p. 27).

A grave error that Kübler-Ross shares with many others is the failure to distinguish between a patient's attitude toward *death* and *dying of cancer.* In a book *On Death and Dying* and a chapter on "Attitudes Toward Death and Dying" few confusions could be more fateful; of course, the prospect of being very slowly tortured to death, of becoming increasingly helpless and a burden to others, is fearful; but it obviously does not follow that the fear of *death* is universal.

Kübler-Ross also fails to note how her data in the chapter on "Attitudes Toward Death and Dying" point to cultural conditioning—and to the inauthenticity of those who minister to the patients. They carry on an elaborate, institutionalized ritual of deception. She mentions that "all the patients knew about their terminal illness anyway, whether they were explicitly told or not" (p. 31) but adds that they were usually not told the whole truth, and that the doctors rationalized their own deception by claiming "that their patients do not want to know the truth, that they never ask for it, and that they believe all is well" (p. 32). Her evidence is abundant and clear, but does not seem to budge her own dogmatic faith. "I approached him hesitantly and asked him simply, 'How sick are you?' 'I am full of cancer . . .' was his answer. The problem was that nobody ever asked a simple straightforward question. They mistook his grim look as a closed door; in fact, their own anxiety prevented them from finding out" (p. 35). But seven pages later she repeats her dogma: "Since in our unconscious mind we are all immortal, it is almost inconceivable for us to acknowledge that we too have to face death."

The point is not to find fault with an author who has done

her best to humanize the care of the dying. She deserves our respect and gratitude. But her data show much more than she realizes and expose forcefully not only the *inhumanity* of legions of people who minister to the dying but also their *dishonesty*. Kübler-Ross, like many other authors, makes much of the self-deception of the dying, of their inauthentic faith that they are *not* dying. But she also shows, without seeming to notice it, that the whole project of prolonging the lives of the terminally ill reeks of the inauthentic faith that the patient is not about to die. Not only is the patient systematically deceived *with words*, but all the tremendous effort and expense directed toward him make sense only on the assumption that the patient is *not* about to die. If he occasionally comes to believe that he is not about to die, it is scarcely reasonable to blame *him* or to seek an explanation in terms of Kübler-Ross's psychoanalytic dogma. After all, one is generally said to show the seriousness of one's beliefs by one's *actions* and by how much money one is willing to put up for them. If people spend thousands of dollars on one's hospital care, it stands to reason that one is led to think, at least sometimes, that one is *not* about to die.

It has become fashionable to play with the idea that the "insane" are really sane while our society is insane. My point is not so Manichaean. From the obvious fact that our society is insane in some ways it hardly follows that the "insane" are really sane. In our society some dogmas about death and suicide that are part of the legacy of Christianity, and as unsupported by empirical evidence as most other Christian dogmas, are still very widely accepted. There are other dogmas that come from other sources, including Freud. The point is not to blame either Christianity or Freud. Those who did not know it before can learn from Alvarez how eager many early Christians were to die a martyr's death—so much so that a callous Roman proconsul did not know how to manage such huge numbers and wrote back to Rome for advice. Not long afterward, Christian attitudes changed. But our concern here is not with the *origin* of dogmas but rather with the ways in which to this day unsupported articles of faith lead to irrational behavior, large-scale deception, and inhumanity.

Kübler-Ross is exceptionally humane, but even she shares this irrationality. She is superb when she derides the nurses who are reluctant to ease the intolerable pain of the dying with an injection because they are afraid that the patient, on the threshold of death, might become an addict. But take, as a final example, the twenty-page interview she prints in her fourth chapter. It is far from clear why she should include all those pages; they certainly do not prove any point she might wish to make. But they allow us once again to look behind the scenes and see how an author who wants to be nonjudgmental keeps passing highly irrational judgments on a patient who is far more rational than the doctor and the chaplain, who come across as feeling superior and rather in a hurry.

In the end, I remain quite unconvinced that the fear of death is universal. I have stated my own very different views in the chapter on "Death" in *The Faith of a Heretic* (1961).[3] But being a philosopher who lacks the wealth of concrete experience that so many doctors and nurses have, I naturally wonder sometimes whether there is evidence that proves me wrong. The two books considered here provide a great deal of evidence to show that it is quite possible to face one's own death without fear, although the widespread disbelief in this possibility makes it harder than it need be. Moreover, our hospital system seems to be predicated on the irrational and vicious notion that death is unnatural and must be fought and postponed as long as at all possible, no matter how much dishonesty and inhumanity this may involve. Frederick the Great is said to have sent his soldiers into battle, saying sardonically, *Kerls, wollt ihr denn ewig leben?*—"What is the

3. Garden City, N.Y.: Doubleday, 1961. Anchor Books paperback, 1963.

matter with you guys? Do you want to live forever?" Our
attitudes toward war have changed, but our modern attitude
toward death is not necessarily more humane. It is insane to
try to make the terminally ill live forever, and to try to make
them believe, by word and deed, that they will. It would be far
better to discuss with them rationally what the options are and
to give those who have the wish to do so the means to live well
as long as that is possible and then to make a dignified end of
it all. Women have won the right to have an abortion. It is
high time to win everyone's right to end his own life without
futile humiliation, torture, and indignity. Here, as so often,
humanity depends on honesty.

Index

Abstraction, faculty of, 151–56
Alexander of Hales, 122
Alvarez, A.: on artists' suicides, 69; *The Savage God: A Study of Suicide*, 235–36, 238
Analysis, existential. *See* Psychiatry
Andersen, Hans Christian: *The Emperor's New Clothes*, 7 and n4
Anxiety: definition of, 217–18
Archimedes, 131
Aristotle, 131
Art: dream and fantasy related to, 3, 27–32; and psychoanalysis, 3

Bateson, G., 58
Bauer, Felice, 64, 65
Beauvoir, Simone de: on creativity, 70; on use of words, 55
Bergmann, Sven Arne: on Strindberg, 73–96
Binswanger, Ludwig, 127; "Case of Ellen West," 206; "The Human Being in Psychiatry," 141
Bleuler, Eugen, 142
Bonaventure: *Itinerarium Mentis ad Deum*, 122
Bosse, Harriet. *See* Strindberg, Harriet Bosse
Boszormenyi-Nagy, Ivan: on Freud, 192; guilt theory of, 222–24; relational therapy, 224–33; *Invisible Loyalties*, 223
Bowen, Murray, 226
Brecht, Bertolt, 67–68
Bremond, Henri: *Histoire littéraire du sentiment religieux*, 101
Brentano, Franz, 128
Broch, Hermann, 45
Brod, Max, 63

Buber, Martin, 191, 207, 208, 212, 221, 225, 228, 229; guilt theory of, 200–01, 224, 230; healing through meeting, 194–97, 201, 205–06; Rogers's dialogue with, 209–11, 214; Trüb influenced by, 198–200; "Healing through Meeting," 197, 205–06; *I and Thou*, 201, 226; *The Knowledge of Man*, 194, 230; "The Psychologizing of the World," 222
Burnham, Donald L.: schizophrenia studies by, 73–74; on Strindberg, 73–96
Butler, Samuel: *Erewhon*, 175

Calvin, John, 131–32
Cappadocian order, 108
Catherine of Siena, 109
Childhood: developmental factors of, 173–89; infantile hallucination, 157–58; infantile imagery, 147; liberative, creative forces of, 51–53, 56; reflected in artistic creativity, 21, 23, 54–55
Chomsky, Noam, 150, 160; and language competence, 152–53; innatism of, 151
Cloud of the Unknowing, The, 109, 110 n16
Communism, 174
Copernicus, Nicolaus, 131–32

Daseinsanalyse. See Psychiatry, existential analysis
Death: artists' suicides, 69; current books on, 235–39; dishonesty about, 238–40; recognition of, 193
Delacroix, H.: *Etudes sur l'histoire et la psychologie des grands mystiques chrétiens*, 115 n34

Psychology, 42, 47, 50; Christianity and, 108; general themes of, 129; psychological novel and, 12, 45; unconscious self and, 103–04
Psychotherapy: family relational, 222–33; healing through meeting, 194–222
Ptolemy, 131
Puente, Luis de la: on concept of the soul, 113 n28

Quakers, 194

Rapaport, D., 147, 157, 164; and levels of representation, 154 n3
Religion: categories of, 101; concepts of the soul and, 105–25; scientific revolt against biblical authority, 129, 131–32; selfhood related to, 102–05
Repression: Freud's concepts of, 19–20, 27, 32; theories of, 42–43
Rhymes: child's creative use of, 52
Richard of St. Victor: on mystical ecstasy, 112 and n24
Ricoeur, Paul; on Freud's relation of dreams and fantasies to art and literature, 3–33; relates psychoanalysis and language, 149–50; Freud and Philosophy, 6 n3, 31 n9, 149
Rogers, Carl R.: Buber's dialogue with, 209–11, 214; healing through meeting, 206–11; On Becoming a Person, 207; "The Loneliness of Contemporary Man," 206
Rohde, Erwin, 107
Romantic era; literary concepts of, 38–39, 42–49 passim
Russell, Bertrand, 136; on modern science related to man, 130
Ruusbroec, Jan van: and mystical experience, 109, 123–24

St. Augustine, 108; memory theory of, 121–22; mysticism of, 111–12; De Trinitate XIV, 121
St. John of the Cross: and imaginary vision, 105, 114–16 passim, 118–19, 121; soul concept of, 109, 112; The Dark Night of the Soul, 112, 119
St. Paul, 108
St. Teresa: and imaginary vision, 115 and n32, 33, 35, 36, 117, 118, 119 n46; on the soul, 109, 112–13
Saussure, F. de: and arbitrariness, 164 n6; and linguistic signs, 152
Scaramelli, Giovanni: Directorio mistico, 113 n28
Schelling, Friedrich, 103
Schiller, Johann: "On Spontaneous and Reflective Poetry," 48, 49
Schizophrenia: and need-fear dilemma, 73–74. See also Strindberg, August
Schlegel, Friedrich, 48
Scholasticism: scientific revolt against, 129
Schopenhauer, Arthur: The World as Will and Idea, 49
Science, modern: emergence of, 129–37
Self-destruction: artistic, creative liberation related to, 57–70; drugs and, 54
Selfhood: religion related to, 102–05; religious concepts of the soul, 105–25
Sexuality: Freud's concepts of, 7, 13, 31–32
Shakers, 194
Shakespeare, William: Freud's study of Hamlet, 10–11, 16, 31
Shankara, 122
Singer, M. T., 58
Skinner, B. F., 151, 153, 208
Smith, Joseph H.: on absent object's genealogical stages, 145–46; on absent object's meaning, 148–49; on abstraction function, 151–56; on arbitrariness of signifiers, 153–55, 161–64; on conceptual and symbolic modes of thought organization, 165–67; on imperative and nonimperative modes of thought organization, 164–65, 167; on nonimperative mentation and play, 161–64; on primary and secondary